D1563589

The Jossey-Bass Health Care Series brings together the most current information and ideas in health care from the leaders in the field. Titles from the Jossey-Bass Health Care Series include these essential health care resources:

After Restructuring: Empowerment Strategies at Work in America's Hospitals, *Thomas G. Rundall, David B. Starkweather, Barbara R. Norrish*

Agility in Health Care: Strategies for Mastering Turbulent Markets, *Steven L. Goldman, Carol B. Graham*

At Risk in America: The Health and Health Care Needs of Vulnerable Populations in the United States, *Lu Ann Aday*

Clinical Integration: Strategies and Practices for Organized Delivery Systems, *Mary Tonges*

Competitive Managed Care: The Emerging Health Care System, *John D. Wilkerson, Kelly J. Devers, Ruth S. Givens, Editors*

Creating Excellence in Crisis Care: A Guide to Effective Training and Program Designs, *Lee Ann Hoff, Kazimiera Adamowski*

Creating the New American Hospital: A Time for Greatness, *V. Clayton Sherman*

Curing Health Care: New Strategies for Quality Improvement, *Donald M. Berwick, A. Blanton Godfrey, Jane Roessner*

Customer Service in Health Care: A Grassroots Approach to Creating a Culture of Excellence, *Kristin Baird*

Designing and Conducting Health Surveys: Second Edition, *Lu Ann Aday*

Error Reduction in Health Care: A Systems Approach to Improving Patient Safety, *Patrice L. Spath, Editor*

Grading Health Care: The Science and Art of Developing Consumer Scorecards, *Pamela P. Hanes, Merwyn R. Greenlick*

Health Behavior and Health Education: Theory Research and Practice, *Karen Glanz, Frances Marcus Lewis, Barbara K. Rimer, Editors*

Health Care 2010: The Forecast, The Challenge, *Institute for the Future*

Health Care in the New Millennium: Vision, Values, and Leadership, *Ian Morrison*

Honoring Patient Preferences: A Guide to Complying with Multicultural Patient Requirements, *Anne Knights Rundle, Maria Carvalho, Mary Robinson, Editors*

Improving Clinical Practice: Total Quality Management and the Physician, *David Blumenthal, Ann C. Scheck, Editors*

Managing Patient Expectations: The Art of Finding and Keeping Loyal Patients, *Susan Keane Baker*

Medical Staff Peer Review, Revised Edition: Motivation and Performance in the Era of Managed Care, *Daniel A. Lang, MD*

Physician Profiling: A Source Book for Health Care Administrators, *Neill F. Piland, Kerstin B. Lynam, Editors*

Profiting from Quality: Outcomes Strategies for Medical Practice, *Steven Isenberg, Richard Gliklich*

Raising Standards in American Health Care: Best People, Best Practices, Best Results, *V. Clayton Sherman*

Remaking Health Care in America: Building Organized Delivery Systems, *Stephen M. Shortell, Robin R. Gillies, David A. Anderson, Karen Morgan Erickson, John B. Mitchell*

Remaking Medicaid: Managed Care for the Public Good, *Stephen M. Davidson, Stephen A. Somers, Editors*

Restructuring Chronic Illness Management: Best Practices and Innovations in Team-Based Treatment, *Jon B. Christianson, Ruth A. Taylor, David J. Knutson*

Status One: Breakthroughs in High Risk Population Health Management, *Samuel Forman, Matthew Kelliher*

Strategic Leadership in Medical Groups: Navigating Your Strategic Web, *John D. Blair, Myron D. Fottler*

Technology and the Future of Health Care: Preparing for the Next 30 Years, *David Ellis*

The 21st Century Health Care Leader, *Roderick W. Gilkey, Editor and The Center for Healthcare Leadership, Emory University School of Medicine*

The New Health Partners: Renewing the Leadership of Physician Practice, *Stephen E. Prather*

Through the Patient's Eyes: Understanding and Promoting Patient-Centered Care, *Margaret Gerteis, Susan Edgman-Levitan, Jennifer Daley, Thomas L. Delbanco*

Total Customer Satisfaction: A Comprehensive Approach for Health Care Providers, *Stephanie G. Sherman, V. Clayton Sherman*

Total Quality in Healthcare: From Theory to Practice, *Ellen J. Gaucher, Richard J. Coffey*

Health Data Quest

Jill Lenk Schilp
Roy E. Gilbreath

Health Data Quest

How to Find and Use Data for Performance Improvement

Jossey-Bass Publishers • San Francisco

Jossey-Bass books and products are available through most
bookstores. To contact Jossey-Bass directly, call (888) 378-2537,
fax to (800) 605-2665, or visit our website at www.josseybass.com.

Substantial discounts on bulk quantities of Jossey-Bass books are
available to corporations, professional associations, and other
organizations. For details and discount information, contact the
special sales department at Jossey-Bass.

Manufactured in the United States of America on Lyons Falls
Turin Book. This paper is acid-free and 100 percent totally
chlorine-free.

Library of Congress Cataloging-in-Publication Data

Health data quest: how to find and use data for performance
improvement.—1st ed.
        p.   cm.
      Edited by Jill Lenk Schilp and Roy E. Gilbreath.
      Includes bibliographical references and index.
      ISBN 0-7879-4155-7
      1. Medical informatics. 2. Medical records—Data processing.
   3. Outcome assessment (Medical care)—Data processing.
   4. Medicine—Quality control—Data processing. I. Schilp, Jill
   Lenk, 1947– II. Gilbreath, Roy E., 1953–
   R858 .H347 2000
   362.1'068'4—dc21   99-050829

FIRST EDITION
HB Printing   10 9 8 7 6 5 4 3 2 1

Contents

List of Figures

Preface

This book is about finding and using information to measure and create health care value. The chapters weave together a tapestry of models, issues, and tools to meet these ends.

Looking for integrated health care data and turning these data into information is like being a *data detective*. It is an adventure. It is also difficult work, but when providers follow the right clues and know how to read and use them, they solve what we call the value equation.

The ability to manage health care data efficiently and turn them into information that proves (or disproves) the value equation is a significant competitive advantage in health care today. The success of a health care organization depends on effective sharing of critical information and the formulation of integrated knowledge by the community of practice acting collaboratively.

Providers and purchasers of care demand valid and reliable measurements, or metrics, that show care is high quality and cost effective. This demand for information can often overwhelm organizational resources. New, more efficient models for gathering data and producing usable information are essential. An integrated and efficient approach is needed to link clinical and cost outcomes of care, measuring both quality and cost across the entire continuum. Skillful data *touring*, *farming*, and *exploring* are required to excavate the true gems of data that reveal outcomes of care.

It is a rare administrator or clinician who has not wondered why it takes so long to produce performance data. However, clinical knowledge workers in search of these integrated data face significant challenges. They must determine what data they really need, distinguishing the important from the unimportant. Then they need to devise efficient ways to find these data and to organize the flow of information. They need resources and tools to accomplish these tasks.

This book will help both clinicians and administrators understand the present information system environment and identify what other organizations are doing to make the best use of the data available. Lessons from others can help each organization create its own information processing system to support its knowledge workers.

This is not a book about *what* to do. It is about *how* to do it. Moreover, outcome management literature typically focuses on how to develop and design health care outcome studies. This book focuses on how clinical knowledge workers can integrate and use data.

We address key issues confronting clinical knowledge workers and major stakeholders in performance improvement. A health care organization must determine what data it really needs to be competitive. By focusing only on the data that matter, the organization can reduce and eventually eliminate non-value-added data capture. Communities of practice need to learn through common experience what information system architecture will best prepare them for the emerging complexity of health care in the twenty-first century.

Audience

Health Data Quest has been written for the broad range of organizations and providers who desire to create and document superior value in health care services. Confronted with increased demands for data describing the clinical and financial outcomes of care, providers and organizations need a guide to finding these data.

This book is also a practical reference on specific topics for selected target audiences.

The first part of the book addresses the information knowledge community and will interest individuals who conduct performance improvement studies, including clinicians, quality managers, and data analysts. Those who are looking to make better use of data to improve care will be particularly interested in the issues and case studies described in the second part of the book.

In addition to being a resource for providers and organizations, *Health Data Quest* is a practical reference for students and instructors in medical informatics, quality management, and performance improvement. Graduate students in health care administration, nursing administration, and medical economics increasingly recognize that the ability to manage health information is a core competency for tomorrow's health care leaders and providers.

Overview of the Contents

Our organizing theme is the complexity of the environment and issues that support and drive data discovery in health care. Part One explains where data discovery occurs; Part Two offers issues and examples of how it occurs.

Part One describes the information knowledge community both practically and conceptually. Beginning with why organizations need data and how they assess the data they have and need, it then moves to discussions of the clinical knowledge community and its technical infrastructure. It includes chapters on clinical systems and medical management.

Chapter One describes the demand for value that confronts the clinical knowledge worker and the quest to find data that demonstrate the value of health care. Performance improvement requires measurement of value. Quality managers and providers must search for appropriate metrics. The value equation, a framework for linking clinical and cost outcomes, is introduced here.

Chapter Two explains how to conduct a data inventory and select indicators of performance. These and the other tools described here are essential for finding and using the data needed to measure value in today's managed care environment and for reducing non-value-added data collection and analysis.

Chapter Three presents a conceptual model of information system processing and introduces the reader to the role of the clinical knowledge worker in performance improvement. It defines a knowledge-based enterprise as a self-organizing, learning, adaptive system characterized by a customer focus, standardized vocabulary, and reduction in non-value-added activities.

Building on this conceptual model, Chapter Four introduces an information technology infrastructure to support data analysis and data mining by clinical knowledge workers. We also review the trends in the evolution of the information processing organization to help the reader understand the challenging context clinical knowledge workers confront in their journeys of discovery.

Chapter Five builds on Chapter Four by reviewing different types of clinical systems, including practice management systems, clinical document systems, workflow and decision support systems, severity systems, patient-provider systems, and managed care information systems. It closes with a discussion of systems analysis, design, and implementation. The information is presented in the context of the new provider-sponsored coordinated care organizations that are developing, although it is relevant to other contexts as well.

Chapter Six proposes several tactics for information-based medical management: physician support alliances, interdisciplinary clinical work teams, project management, clinical measurement and quantitative analysis, benchmarking, and communication and innovation. The chapter's overview of the concepts of medical management is also preparation for part two, as it provides some considerations for practical applications such as physician profiling and drilling down in data that can ultimately lead to quality improvements.

We turn in Part Two to the real world of the clinical knowledge community, presenting key issues as they are reflected in the work of data pioneers. The common theme of Part Two is that information is the foundation of the knowledge community. The case studies and other discussions of practical issues in this section show how today's clinical knowledge workers pursue their data quests.

Chapter Seven reviews the legal issues in health care data management. The sensitivity of health care data and some methods for achieving the precarious balance between access and protection of privacy are explained, and issues in developing data policy are explored.

Adjustment of health care data to reflect the severity of patient illness fully often has financial consequences for health care organizations. Chapter Eight discusses the issues related to severity adjustment and the limitations of financially derived data in this area. Using the team approach to select a severity of illness system enhances collaboration and consensus and can result in a system aligned with business processes.

Chapter Nine proposes that clinical integration of performance improvement data is not just a tool for improvement, it is improvement. Clinical integration requires intense and dynamic patterns of communication, innovation, and consistent processes. Maintaining a flow of information for real-time decision making and support of clinically integrated care delivery models is described as a key performance improvement strategy for the collaborative community.

The case study in Chapter Ten illustrates the challenge of integrating enterprisewide health care information. It reviews practical changes a large health care system made to improve transcription services, chart management, and clinical abstracting.

Chapter Eleven presents approaches to *drilling down* to find integrated performance improvement indicators. This case study shows how quality managers used business applications software to increase data support for their fast-track continuous quality improvement effort.

A clinical pathway assists a team of clinicians to focus on key variables. Chapter Twelve addresses a question asked by most organizations involved in the development and implementation of these pathways: Did our pathway work? The author of this chapter shows how case managers analyzed the root cause of variation in a clinical therapy and demonstrates the clinical integration of disparate data sources in a health care system.

The case study in Chapter Thirteen shows how a balanced scorecard that integrates clinical, financial, and customer service data is analogous to a visual snapshot of an organization's performance. The authors of this study deal with the challenge of communicating this tool to a wide audience while balancing the need to protect sensitive data.

Knowledge improves care only when it is applied. Chapter Fourteen presents a physician's perspective on successful methods of presenting performance information to clinicians. The author suggests creating a *climate of discovery* and describes critical factors that influence clinician acceptance of data.

The final chapter summarizes the common themes seen in the environment, issues, and tools of clinical knowledge workers. It analyzes lessons learned and looks toward the future architecture and support systems of health care data and the trends in that data.

This book illustrates the search for integrated data. A pattern is apparent in the way clinical knowledge workers do their discovery work. It starts with data discovery or sleuthing and proceeds in iterative, drill-down steps. Clinical knowledge workers use an innovative process of discovery and adaptation in their quest for integrated data. Present information systems environments support this process with varying degrees of success.

Organizations can learn from the successful initiatives of others and create their own tools for successful data quests. The search for information to use to improve care is an important but challenging endeavor for today's clinical knowledge worker.

Explore the following chapters and discover how to find and use integrated data for performance improvement in health care. Be a data detective.

December 1999

Jill Lenk Schilp
Dallas, Texas
Roy E. Gilbreath
Atlanta, Georgia

Acknowledgments

We wish to acknowledge the efforts of the contributors and other performance improvement analysts, clinical knowledge workers in the health care organizations who shared their data quests with us. We are also indebted to the health care organizations—the Baylor Health Care System and the Promina Health Care System—that nurtured us and created in us the passion for improvement and spirit of inquiry that provided the stimulus for this endeavor.

We owe special thanks to Andy Pasternack, senior health editor at Jossey-Bass Inc., Publishers, who provided much wisdom and patient counsel to us in our journey, and to Cynthia Orticio, who provided expert help in the manuscript preparation.

Finally, special thanks to George Schilp, who so faithfully provided technical support and desktop services.

Jill Lenk Schilp
Roy E. Gilbreath

The Authors

Roy E. Gilbreath is a practicing general internist with twenty years of clinical experience. He received his MD degree from the University of Miami and completed his internal medicine residency at Walter Reed Army Medical Center. After serving six years in the U.S. Army, he practiced in California, Texas, and Georgia. He later received an MBA degree from the University of Nevada-Reno, and he has held several physician-administrator positions over the past six years. He is currently vice president of system clinical services with Promina Gwinnett Health System. Gilbreath's interests are in the areas of performance improvement, clinical information management and informatics, clinical leadership, and managed care. He received the 1998 Healthcare Information and Management Systems Society (HIMSS) Article of the Year award for his essay "Provider-Sponsored Coordinated Care Organizations: Designing Systems for Patient Centered Care" (reprinted in this book as Chapter Five).

Jill Lenk Schilp is a registered nurse with over twenty years' experience in nursing and performance improvement. She received her BS degree in nursing from Seton Hall University and her MS degree in nursing from Texas Woman's University. She is a certified professional in health care quality and teaches courses in information systems for health care in the graduate program at Texas Woman's University in Dallas. Schilp currently works with VHA, Inc., developing and implementing clinical effectiveness programs. She also has a special interest in performance improvement and using integrated health care data to improve care.

The Contributors

Donna Bowers is director of health information management at Baylor University Medical Center in Dallas.

Patricia Driscoll is associate professor of health care administration at Texas Woman's University and an attorney in private practice in Dallas.

Judy Lawing is director of coordinated care at Promina Gwinnett Health System in Lawrenceville, Georgia.

Susan McBride is director of outcome management at Texas Health Resources in Dallas.

LaVone Neal is vice president of decision support services and financial analysis for the Baylor Health Care System in Dallas.

Bonita A. Pilon is professor for the practice of nursing and associate dean, school of nursing, at Vanderbilt University, Nashville, Tennessee, and has consulted internationally on quality improvement, clinical pathways, and case management.

Annette Rowton is vice president for clinical outcomes with Texas Health System in Dallas.

Stephen Ryter is corporate medical director at Health Care Horizons, Inc., in Albuquerque, New Mexico. He is board certified in pediatrics, a fellow of the American College of Pediatrics, and a member of the American College of Physician Executives.

Jennifer Walker is management engineer for the Baylor Health Care System in Dallas.

Health Data Quest

Part One

The Information Knowledge Community

Part One introduces the present demand for health care data and describes the information knowledge community in which these data must be collected, integrated, and transformed into information to improve care.

Chapter One

Why Do Organizations Need Data?

The demand for health care value creates an increased need for integrated measurements of clinical and cost outcomes. This chapter explores internal and external needs for integrated data and the challenge this presents to the clinical knowledge worker faced with separate islands of information.

The impact of the changing health care landscape is significant for outcomes management and quality improvement. The demand for value in clinical services has never been greater. Payers and patients want proof of the value of health care services, with measures of both quality and cost effectiveness. Health care systems and clinicians need to find innovative ways to deliver high-quality care at a lower cost. Their challenge is to treat patients at the point in the continuum of care where the value is the greatest, providing the right care at the right time in the right place and for the right cost. As a result their need for specific, high-quality data has dramatically increased. Providers need integrated, easily accessible, valid, and reliable data about care delivered at all points in the health care continuum. Furthermore, a great opportunity exists to differentiate health care systems and physician groups on the basis of their service, quality outcomes, and cost effectiveness of care.

Although most health care organizations have data, their real challenge is to find and effectively use the information that will create and document value. If organizations are to do an effective job of developing the knowledge community and knowledge workers, they must minimize non-value-added data retrieval, storage, and analysis. The ability to find and use integrated data about clinical care across the entire continuum is key to surviving and thriving in the new health care environment.

Who Wants Data and Why?

Health care organizations are besieged by an avalanche of requests for information from a variety of internal and external groups and organizations. Analysis and reporting of clinical care appropriateness, process, and utilization and also of outcomes and illness severity are needed to meet regulatory demands. Integrated health care information is needed to support marketing efforts, satisfy regulatory requirements, comply with managed care contracts, and document value to purchasers of care. Effective marketing of health care services requires benchmarking against the services of other providers and comparison of data to data in national subject-oriented repositories. Purchasers increasingly require outcomes reporting that can be used as report cards, or performance profiles, for both institutions and providers and that documents superior value for the health care dollar.

Not long ago, clinical and financial shops rarely combined their data. They virtually spoke different languages. The measurement of value in health care now demands that clinical and financial measurements, or metrics, be integrated.

Clinical value exists in relation to both quality and cost (Figure 1.1). Value and cost are inversely proportional: if cost goes up, value goes down; if cost goes down, value goes up. Quality and value are directly proportional: if quality goes up, value goes up; if quality goes down, value goes down. Actions that decrease cost increase clinical value. Efforts that increase quality increase clinical value. If costs go down but quality also decreases, value decreases. The basic principle of this value equation is that both quality and cost drive health care value. The financial analyst and clinical analyst now solve the *value equation* together.

Figure 1.1. The Value Equation.

$$\text{Value} = \frac{\text{Clinical Quality} + \text{Customer Service}}{\text{Cost}}$$

Process improvement requires integrated information—a combination of clinical, service, quality, and financial data. Examples of clinical data are rates of mortality, infection, unscheduled readmission to the hospital, unscheduled return to surgery, and operative deaths, as well as measures of appropriateness of care and of long-term functional status after treatment. Patient satisfaction scores are one form of data describing service quality. Financial data include cost and charge per case, length of stay and utilization information, and total revenue. These data are examined for trends and also used for comparison and benchmarking. Health care systems and hospitals vary greatly in their ability to produce this information.

Internal Data Requirements

Internal customers of a health care enterprise need integrated clinical and financial data to support continuous improvement efforts, indexing of patient illness severity, monitoring of procedure appropriateness, measurement of clinical outcomes, and resource management. Examples of information required are outcomes, appropriateness, and cost of care; access to care; resource consumption; service quality; illness severity; and process variation. In addition, performance monitoring that aggregates data on functional status after discharge is necessary for the competitive health enterprise. Health care organizations also need to assess customer service through measures of patient satisfaction and to compare these data with those of comparable organizations.

To understand variation in practice patterns, quality improvement teams require data about the processes of care. A key step in process improvement is the identification of an ideal path of care, or *pathway*, for patients with similar needs. Identification and analysis of perceived better practice then provides a mechanism for extending the delivery of proven high-value patterns of care across a larger patient population and for better quantifying and documenting high-value care.

Hospital executives often discover, to their surprise, that external organizations are reporting more data about their hospital's performance than the hospital's internal systems are presently reporting. In this environment, hospitals must identify the information system architecture that can provide internal performance reports that are more current, relevant, and complete than publicly available data sets.

Provider Profiling

Provider profiles, or report cards, compare the performance over time of individual physicians, groups, or departments to an established norm for one or more clinical or financial indicators. Profiling data may be used for performance improvement, credentialing, and quality assurance.

Profiles can be valuable tools for performance improvement if they are designed properly. The success of clinician profiling in meeting its objectives depends on three factors: the confidence of the clinicians in the validity of the data; appropriate treatment of data within the profiles; and appropriate adjustment of the data for the severity of illness of the patient population. Clinicians have confidence in data that are accurate, relevant, timely, and adequately adjusted for severity. Appropriate treatment of data includes comparing physicians, hospitals, or departments with homogeneous populations and constructing profiles to provide characteristics that are useful and valid. Caution is necessary when making assumptions about provider performance when one has not considered all the variables that may affect that performance.

The source for profiling data determines that information's relative ability to accurately reflect a complete clinical picture of the patient and his or her care. Most publicly available profiling is based on administrative data, which are more widely available and less expensive to produce than clinical data. However, claims-based, or administrative, data may not reflect the complete clinical picture. Data derived from clinical systems can provide risk and severity adjustments not captured elsewhere. The issues surrounding the use of administrative data as a source for clinical profiling are discussed in Chapter Eight.

Crossing the Continuum

Clinical integration is the extent to which patient care activities are coordinated across the levels of care to increase the probability of maximum value to the patient. It is the degree to which preventive, diagnostic, and therapeutic processes are delivered to the patient in order to achieve optimal clinical outcomes for both individual patients and aggregate populations and to ensure smooth transitions across time (Tonges, 1998, p. 3). Clinical integration of services across a continuum is a defining characteristic of integrated health care delivery systems (Conrad, 1993; Shortell, Gillies, Anderson, Mitchell, & Morgan, 1993; Shortell, Gillies, Anderson, Erickson, & Mitchell, 1996). Clinical integration requires integrated data.

High-value care is seamless, but most journeys through the health care system are fragmented, less than efficient, and characterized by costly delays and customer dissatisfaction. A patient experiencing one episode of illness may require care at several different levels of intensity and at several different delivery sites. For example, a cardiovascular patient may enter the health care system through a well-patient examination, where only education or assessment of health risk status is performed. Results of the examination may reveal the need for diagnostics, such as radiology or laboratory tests. Abnormal results may occur. The patient must now access the health system as an outpatient to investigate these results. Sometimes he or she may need hospitalization, an emergency room visit, or an intensive care unit stay. A cardiac patient can move from a less-invasive to a more-invasive procedure during one inpatient encounter with care. Following the patient's acute-care encounter, some conditions may require further treatment at home. The ability of a provider to guide the patient and family through each of these levels of care determines both the quality and cost effectiveness of that episode of illness.

To evaluate clinical value the entire episode of illness must be measured, not just a single encounter. For the patient with coronary artery disease the entire course of treatment, from risk intervention to first symptomatic episodes through hospitalization and later bypass surgery, must be examined. The cost outcomes of the bypass surgery are an incomplete measure of outcome. The true value of treatment is analyzed through integrated clinical, financial, patient satisfaction, and functional status data.

As this scenario demonstrates, integrated data from a variety of care sites and levels of care are needed to measure, monitor, and improve care. Many of the data needed today reside in disparate information systems. Merging of several data sources is necessary to study disease management across the continuum. Data must be retrieved from physicians' offices, severity adjustment systems, and inpatient and outpatient pharmacies and laboratories for each encounter. Measures of a patient's functional status and satisfaction with care and access must be integrated. Clinical scenarios surrounding each admission must be available from the database and completely considered.

Clinical Pathways

Clinical pathways are tools that organize and time the interventions of the interdisciplinary team for a patient with a particular case type, subset, or condition (Bergman, 1994). Clinical pathways serve as reminders for caregivers and are individualized, based on the needs of the patient. Variances from the expected path are recorded and analyzed. Clinical pathways can be very effective in analyzing outcomes of care, particularly when data are integrated and variance information is included.

A clinical knowledge worker begins to develop a clinical pathway by identifying a population of interest and selecting and analyzing specific indicators of cost or quality. The path may describe interventions such as preadmission counseling, inpatient visits, cardiac rehabilitation, and postoperative visits. The relationship between the patient's path of care and longitudinal functional status in terms of pain and role function may be investigated. Particularly when there is variance, the analyst may decide that further investigation is needed and begin an iterative process of discovery and exploration of possible reasons for variance. By relating these clinical data to cost and utilization data, the value equation can be determined. The goal is to determine the most effective path of care to achieve the best long-term outcome and the highest degree of function and patient satisfaction. Chapter Twelve presents an example of how nurses used variance data from clinical pathways to investigate an opportunity to improve care.

External Data Requirements

Purchasers of health care require more than general claims such as "we have the best doctors and nurses" or "we have the most modern facility in the state." They require quantitative proof of quality and cost effectiveness. Health care providers, then, need to collect data about their performance and turn those data into information that purchasers can understand. Purchasers are not the only ones seeking such data; governmental regulatory agencies, consumers, and other providers also require evidence of quality. The requirements of external organizations for data vary. However, a number of key health care organizations and initiatives are engaging in early efforts that may set the overall direction for measurement.

JCAHO

Instead of focusing just on processes of care or structural indicators of quality, the Joint Commission on Accreditation of Healthcare Organizations (JCAHO) has begun also using performance measures and outcomes in its accreditation process. This has created a new set of expectations for health care organizations. A comprehensive overview of the JCAHO's current initiatives and standards for indicator development and performance measurement can be found at the JCAHO Website at http://www.jcaho.org.

HEDIS

The Health Plan Employer Data and Information Set (HEDIS) is designed to measure the value of the delivery of care in health plans, focusing on access, membership, utilization, member satisfaction, and quality. HEDIS is becoming more widely used as a measure for documenting health care plan performance and for providing valuable information to purchasers of care and to health plans, to assist them with performance improvement.

Employers and health plans began HEDIS in 1989 to establish certain standardized performance measures that could be used to compare health plans. HEDIS has served as an important catalyst for the development of standardized measurement. Newer versions of HEDIS show even greater promise. A list of the current HEDIS indicators may be found on the NCQA Website at http://www.ncqa.org. Information regarding the history of HEDIS and a description of measurement initiatives of NCQA are also available at this site.

Purchasers

Purchasers want to secure products and services that are cost effective and high quality, and they often define the metrics providers must submit. There are two potential problems with this. First, the measures chosen by purchasers are often quite broad and may not be robust quality indicators. Purchasers keep the measures broad so that a range of providers can report on them and nonclinicians can easily understand them. Second, the best data are often difficult to obtain.

In many communities business groups are working alone or collaboratively to develop more relevant metrics so that more informed purchasing decisions can be made. Purchasers need to identify uniform value indicators. Employers usually need data to educate employees to make informed purchasing decisions as health care consumers, to identify high-value performers from managed care networks, and to identify employee health problems for health improvement programs. These types of efforts by business coalitions have often been catalysts for uniform quality measurement systems in communities. These efforts may also encourage continuous quality improvement and cost effectiveness and may drive a community effort to develop more robust and clinically relevant measures of value.

Value indicators of particular interest to business groups are the cost effectiveness and cost predictability of care, patient satisfaction, clinical quality, and patient health status. The challenge for data integration is the lack of consistent and integrated hospital, physician office, and patient satisfaction data. Available measures are often limited to administrative rather than clinically robust data.

Conclusion

The demand for information to measure health care is growing. Health care value is determined by the relationship between quality and cost. Although finding and using integrated data is often difficult, it is a key to success. Internally, an organization needs data for processes such as performance improvement, provider profiling, and comparative analysis. External individuals and organizations such as purchasers and governmental agencies also require a variety of data. In the next chapter we explore these needs further, and then in Chapters Three and Four we examine the knowledge-based enterprise of the twenty-first century.

Chapter Two

What Data Do Organizations Need?

Performing a Data Needs Assessment

Roy E. Gilbreath

> Like all great detectives, good data sleuths know
> three things: what they already have, what to look
> for, and where to look. This is not as easy as it
> sounds. A *data needs assessment* is a tool to identify
> the data needed by an organization to achieve its
> goals. In addition to discussing the data needs
> assessment, this chapter reviews other tools for a
> successful data quest: the data inventory,
> information gap analysis, and data blueprint.

Most health care organizations today possess a complex infrastructure of departments, committees, functional entities, and professional constituencies. Each of these units generates data. The result is often a collection of uncoordinated indicators of performance, with many different definitions for each data element.

Because searching for data can be time consuming and expensive, data quests must result in the best data to answer the key needs of the organization. At first the increased demand from internal and external individuals and organizations seems to suggest that more is better. In fact, an abundance of data is often the problem. In the midst of the health care data explosion, having many data or the wrong data may be just as problematic as having no data. The real challenge is to search out the data necessary to meet the business needs of the organization and the demands of the public.

A goal of the knowledge community is the reduction of non-value-added work. Health care systems, however, often go to considerable expense to implement clinical information systems only to discover that no real improvements in cost, quality, or time are realized.

The Data Needs Assessment Process

A data needs assessment asks the following questions:

- What are the key business goals and objectives of the organization?
- What are the key business processes?
- Who are the key populations?
- What are the right performance indicators: outcomes? processes? services? cost? health status? access? appropriateness? comparison and benchmarks? Are these indicators important to patients?
- Who needs to know?
- What data does the organization or unit have, and what data does it need?

The following sections explain these questions in more detail.

What Are the Key Business Goals?

Data collection must be integrated with the business plan of the organization. A review of the current business plan; strategic plan; and organizational goals, objectives, and strategies provides a foundation for assessing business needs. This information is usually available in an organization's strategic planning entity or executive offices. The strategic goals of an organization are measurable objectives for a robust and effective program of ongoing, data-driven improvement.

How an organization plans to measure its success defines the key goals for the quality improvement process. For example, if organizational success is defined as having world-class customer service, then this must also be a goal for quality improvement and that goal will require a quest for scores on patient and customer satisfaction surveys. If success is defined as clinical quality that meets or exceeds national benchmarks, other key quality indicators will be required. At the same time, acquisition of the clinical data that make up these quality indicators must be a key business imperative. The organizational strategy must therefore position resources so that people can employ information in support of the organizational vision.

What Are the Key Business Processes?

Data must be collected to measure, monitor, and manage the key business processes. A business process is an activity or set of activities designed to achieve a business goal. Examples of core business processes in health care are the medication administration process, the elective surgery process, the procurement of supplies process, and the performance measurement process.

Who Are the Key Populations?

An organization needs data about the key populations served. An analysis of the high-volume conditions, procedures, and demographic groups served allows the health care organization to target key populations. For example, a hospital whose top-volume service line is obstetrical care should design in-depth data collection on factors related to the care of women's health. At the same time, if an organization is planning strategic growth into a new service line, data on patterns of care and utilization for the relevant population should be collected. A key population may not be limited to patients. Peer review activities and quality assurance needs may require that medical staff be considered a key population.

Once key populations are determined the organization must identify the information needed about them. In the case of patient populations, demographic information such as unique patient identifier, dates and types of services received, and payer may be needed.

What Are the Right Performance Indicators?

Performance indicators are used to measure the quality and cost effectiveness of care. Quality indicators may relate to structures, processes, outcomes, and service. Mammography screening rates are examples of process indicators; breast cancer mortality rates or survival rates are outcomes. Indicators of appropriateness of care measure whether procedures done are necessary. Functional measures show how a patient perceives his or her level of functioning over time. Access indicators measure such variables as waiting time for appointments, drive time to primary care providers, and access to emergency care when needed. Examples of service indicators include waiting times in physicians' offices, patient satisfaction ratings, and the amount of time and personal attention given by caregivers.

Indicators used to evaluate clinical processes and outcomes may include rates for hospital readmissions, admissions to the hospital after outpatient procedures, returns to the operating room, infections, and complications. Other indicators of performance include type and number of encounters with patients, disease management measures, population measures, and preventive service measures.

Several types of indicators may be used for health care improvement: administrative and financial measures and measures of clinical performance, health status, and service and satisfaction. Each can be reported at different levels of aggregation, or groupings—patient, provider, condition, procedure, and organization.

Resource indicators such as severity-adjusted length of stay and costs per case are important value indicators. The interrelationship of cost and quality—the value equation—is a key focus in evaluating clinical value. Negative events such as infections or complications may result in increased resource consumption and longer length of stay. Premature discharge may result in costly readmission to the hospital.

Common disease- and procedure-specific measures, such as wound infection rates in surgery patients, are also used to measure quality. Generic measures, such patients' perceptions of their status at a given point in time, provided via a patient questionnaire, are used to determine general health status. Generic measures are usually supplemented by condition-specific measures because generic measures often do not provide enough clinical detail about each particular type of patient.

Many indicators are procedure specific and rate based—that is, they are expressed in terms of the percentage of times that a procedure was performed on a given population (for example, a hospital might have an X percent cesarean section rate among its obstetrical patients). In some cases, a national standard, or benchmark, may exist that targets a perceived desired rate.

There is currently no universally accepted standard definition of a core set of measurements of health care quality. Many organizations are searching for a consistent set of uniform, cost-effective performance measures that can measure quality with validity, reliability, and sensitivity.

All measures are not created equal. Based on the business needs of the organization and the needs of internal and external customers, only those indicators should be used that can be collected in accord with the key criteria of economy, validity, reliability, and the other attributes of a good measure.

A good performance measure meets the following criteria:

- Validity: in order to be scientifically sound, useful, and accurate, a measure must have validity; it must measure what it is supposed to measure.

- Reliability: a reliable metric measures the attribute consistently over time. That is, different raters using the same measure are likely to get the same results over repeated measurements. Validity and reliability are interrelated. The development of enterprisewide data definitions provides the foundation for data reliability and validity. When Hospital A in a health care system defines a *readmission* as a patient admitted to the hospital within thirty-one days of a previous hospitalization, Hospital B defines it as a patient readmitted to the hospital within thirty-two days of the last admission, and Hospital C defines it as a patient readmitted to the hospital within thirty days of a previous admission for a condition or procedure related to the previous condition for which the patient was admitted, the enterprise's definitions lack precision and consistency and an enterprisewide definition is needed. In addition, even a single data definition may cause difficulties when, as is likely, different data collectors interpret it differently. Common operational data definitions must be developed.

- Accuracy: an accurate measure can be verified. The methods by which data are collected drive data accuracy.

- Timeliness: a good measure is timely. Real-time performance improvement cannot meet its goals when the data it relies on are not timely.

- Relevance: a good measure is relevant to the organization. It reflects the major business strategy goals and objectives and it quantifies the progress made toward meeting them. Measures and data must also matter to the customer.

- Precise definitions: a measure should have a clear, written definition that is not subject to different interpretations. If it is a rate-based indicator, the numerator and denominator will be clearly defined (Joint Commission on Accreditation of Healthcare Organizations, 1999).

- Targeted opportunities: a good measure should target opportunities for improvement and point the way to making those improvements.

- Sensitivity: a measure has to be sensitive enough to discern changes in the attribute it is measuring. Differences between patients are important. Condition-specific measures may be necessary to drive clinical performance improvement.

- Feasibility: a good measure is also feasible to collect. Small organizations may be able to use manual data collection more economically than large organizations. Larger organizations may have more automation available.

- Freedom from bias: a measure should be objective, and objectivity should be built into the process of data collection. Examples of patient factors that may create bias are severity of illness and preexisting health status. An indicator should be adjusted for these factors to the extent possible.

- Ease of understanding: a good measure is simple and easy to understand.

Who Needs to Know?

The next step in the needs assessment is to identify the data needs of the key groups. Review the information needs of each customer, department, or constituency, noting any areas of duplication. Use data flow diagrams to analyze methods of data retrieval, storage, and outputs.

Information about customers' needs can be obtained from department objectives, statements of department visions and scope, professional and regulatory standards that govern the activity of the entity, organizational charts, and patterns of internal and external communication. In a data needs assessment, customers for data should be asked the following questions:

- What information do you need about products and services in your area of responsibility? Ongoing processes of care?

Customer, employee, and physician satisfaction? Managed care contracting? Program evaluation and ongoing quality improvement? Clinical and cost benefits of programs and services?

- What external information requests do you receive?
- Who collects data for you now?
- What data are collected?
- When are data collected?
- What data are reported and to whom?
- How long do you need to keep data?
- Why are these data collected?

Internal performance improvement needs drive internal data requirements. External needs drive external data requirements. The data each department or group interviewed needs for accreditation and certification may be different for each accrediting agency. The results of the data needs assessment yield an overview of the data needs of the entire organization.

What Data Does the Organization or Unit Have, and What Data Does It Need?

The *data inventory*, a systematic search for and classification of the performance improvement data that already exist in an organization, is a key component of the data assessment.

A data inventory frequently reveals an organization to be rich with disparate, uncoordinated pieces of data, only some of which it may need. Traditionally, health care data have been gathered to solve specific business needs. Most of these data have never been integrated into a measurement system that focuses on the key indicators of performance. The goal of the data inventory is to determine the *information gap*—to compare what is needed with what is available. A data inventory must also determine which of the data that are available are actually needed.

The secret to a successful data inventory is knowing where to look. Many individuals and groups in health care organizations need data, so data exist in many places. The three major sources of data for a health care system are usually internal data systems (including financial databases, transaction databases, billing databases, and clinical department databases), purchased data, and public data. These sources include enrollment files, administrative records, clinical information contained in medical records, patient and provider surveys, and data collected by external private organizations and public agencies (McGlynn, Damberg, Kerr, & Shenker, 1998). Data can also be found in business plans, annual reports, and proposals developed for market research and contracting.

Enrollment files contain data generated from health insurance plans and government databases such as those for Medicare and Medicaid. Aggregation of enrollment statistics is important in measuring quality indicators, because these statistics provide a denominator for measuring the health or interventions directed at populations or groups of members with a particular condition. Administrative data resulting from claims or billing processes are widely available in health care organizations. They include encounter-specific data about services provided during the processes of care. If a process or service is billed, it is typically captured in an administrative system. Administrative data are useful in identifying transactions that result from patients' interaction with the health care system and can be used to identify groups of patients who received certain services. Because administrative data lack clinical depth, however, they are of limited usefulness in analyzing some aspects of quality (see Chapter Eight).

Clinical information found in the medical record is a significant source of information for quality improvement. The value of this information depends on the accuracy and completeness of the clinician's documentation. In order to obtain rich clinical information from this source, labor-intensive manual abstraction of information is frequently necessary. The increase in performance profiling is acting as a catalyst for improvement in the documentation and coding practices in health care organizations that recognize that more complete records mean more accurate pictures of their performance.

Committees and task forces in a health care organization frequently collect data. Committees most likely to need and collect clinical or cost effectiveness measures are those charged with strategic planning, infection control, credentialing, quality assurance and quality improvement, utilization management, case management, clinical path development and implementation, peer review, process redesign, drug use evaluation, product evaluation, and customer service.

Most organizations measure some degree of patient satisfaction. This information can be integrated with resource and quality data into overall performance measures and can constitute an important part of demonstration of value.

Tools for the Data Needs Assessment

Two tools are particularly useful in a data needs assessment: a data flow analysis and a data blueprint.

Data Flow Analysis

It is useful to map how the different databases that have data in the inventory communicate with each other. One of the significant problems in collecting data is the absence of linkages among them. Valuable clinical information may reside in stand-alone stores, and a data flow analysis will reveal both where data are shared and where they are not shared, indicating the variety of sources that may need to be tapped.

The Data Blueprint

What quantity of data is enough? Organizations answer this question by comparing the data needs assessment with the data inventory and preparing a *data blueprint*. The blueprint specifies an indicator of performance for each need and the data needed for each indicator (Figure 2.1). The best indicators are those that are of most interest to external and internal payers, those that can double as cost and quality indicators, and those that can be collected with economy and validity. Several indicators have dual utility in that they affect dual aspects of costs of care and quality of care. Examples of dual utility indicators are length of stay, unplanned readmission, and rates of complications and other adverse events. These indicators may be of special value in quality improvement activities and of interest to purchasers of health care. The blueprint also requires the organization to determine data availability and whether concise definitions exist for each data element.

At this point, a clinical knowledge worker preparing a blueprint for a particular performance indicator is confronted with the information gap (Figure 2.2): "I have some data I don't need, and I need data I don't have." Solving the information gap is the essence of the data quest.

Conclusion

Information systems alone do not improve care; they are merely tools that have to be manipulated by clinical knowledge workers. The way to achieve performance improvement is to focus on the information that makes a difference to patient care and to the clinicians who provide that care. To reduce non-value-added work the clinical knowledge worker should spend time looking for only the most valuable data.

Figure 2.1. Data Blueprint for Performance Improvement.

Key aspect of care to be measured _____

Performance indicator (specify numerator/denominator) _____

Data Needed	Population (Specify ICD-9 or CPT Codes)	Data Source	Who Will Perform? Input	Who Will Perform? Output	Who Will Perform? Validity Check	Time to Collect Data and Technical Requirements	Why We Need to Collect Data (Business Case)
		Database (specify):					
		1.					
		2.					
		3.					
		Medical record:					
		Concurrent review:					
		Retro review:					
		Other (specify):					
		1.					
		2.					
		Data cannot be collected (explain):					

All Audiences for Data	Data Period (by Date of Discharge)	Reporting Frequency	Aggregate	
1.	Fiscal year: ___	One time only? ___	Patient ___	Are consistent definitions already available?
2.	Fiscal quarter: ___	Ongoing? ___	Payer ___	If no, specify plan: ___
3.	Calendar year: ___	Quarterly: ___	Provider ___	
4.	Calendar quarter: ___	Monthly: ___	DRG ___	
	Month: ___	Annually: ___	Diagnosis ___	
Approval or releases required:	From ___ to ___	Other: ___	Procedure ___	
1.	(Y/M/D) (Y/M/D)		Unit ___	
2.			Product Line ___	Date plan completed: ___
3.			Other ___	Revised: ___
4.				Target implementation date: ___

Figure 2.2. Finding the Information Gap.

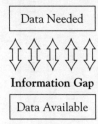

By conducting a data needs assessment and a data inventory, the gap between the data needed and the data on hand is identified. This provides the basis for the search for missing data. Alignment of data collection with the business goals of the organization is key to ensuring benefit.

We now turn in Chapters Three and Four to the information processing environment that supports performance improvement.

Chapter Three

The Health Care Information Processing Environment

A Knowledge-Based Enterprise

Roy E. Gilbreath

Health care is delivered by knowledge-driven communities of practice. The *information processing organization* is the operational implementation of the knowledge-based enterprise. Clinical knowledge workers in search of performance improvement use a process of creative discovery. This chapter presents a conceptual model for the health care information processing organization, describing how a health care information processing organization works, the social environment needed to support the knowledge-based enterprise, and the process of discovery and data mining in performance improvement.

Information processing in health care relies on the collective knowledge of the organization's workers. This knowledge becomes the driving force for defining and continuously refining the organization's core competencies, the critical skills necessary to support the selected products and services. Strategies arise from clear delineation of the core competencies and the value that is to be delivered to the designated customers or market. Furthermore, the knowledge-based enterprise must link critical knowledge resources to accomplish these strategies through high operational performance. This linkage has the effect of nurturing workers with knowledge and expanding organizational creativity through collaboration (Manville & Foote, 1996b).

Knowledge workers, through information sharing and empowerment, use and contribute to the enterprise's knowledge store as they interact with customers and perform duties. As a result, knowledge workers exhibit raised aspirations and enhanced creativity compared to other workers; they also have less risk aversion and territorialism (Manville & Foote, 1996a).

The characteristics of the knowledge-based enterprise, as noted in many industries, are

- A customer service focus
- Formal and informal worker collaboration
- A standardized vocabulary and processes
- A reduction in non-value-added activities
- Integrated outcomes analysis and reporting for the purposes of accountability for value delivered
- Operational and financial linkages
- A self-organizing adaptive system

In addition, many knowledge-based organizations are deploying a management infrastructure to promote their further development. The chief knowledge officer is responsible for creating the appropriate knowledge sharing environment and making the knowledge base available in useful formats. The chief knowledge officer creates resource slack, formulates incentives, and champions performance measurement for the organization. Moreover, the executive leadership fosters a culture of emergent control, so that innovation and creativity arise from collaborating agents within the knowledge-based enterprise.

Information Delivery

The free flow of information is critical to the success of the health care knowledge-based enterprise and information processing organization. The *management information system* (MIS) concept has recently given way to the *information delivery system* concept. Historically, health care information systems have been administratively and financially focused, with a departmental orientation and a return on investment benefits analysis. Useful operational or point of care information systems were lacking.

The information delivery system has been metaphorically referred to as an *ecosystem*, a system that is surviving within the environmental constraints through the evolutionary and emergent interaction of a community of workers (Inmon, Imhoff, & Sousa, 1998).

The information delivery system assists users in the formation of these communities of practice and enables them to share knowledge through *pull* as opposed to *push*. A *community of practice* is a group of agents within a given domain with similar tasks and goals with regard to customer needs and outcomes. A pull mechanism, or process, is one that cues the next interaction. A push process relies on the next person in the process to originate the need for task accomplishment. Ideally in the information delivery system, accountability for critical performance measures is an incentive to collaboration.

The information delivery system enables a community of workers to follow their knowledge-driven inspirations through real-time analysis of historical data. It supplies the tools for workers to analyze previous experiences and to support innovations.

The success of this information ecosystem depends on the effective and efficient sharing of critical information and on a conception of knowledge through collaboration. Hoarding, territorialism, unique vocabularies, diverse agendas, and unaligned incentives are a disadvantage to the organization in this process.

The complexities of today's environment demand a flexible and adaptable health care delivery system. Patients are demanding improved access. Employers want accountability for high quality and error-free delivery of health services. Payers are requiring even greater cost savings with lower prices and competitive bidding. As financing mechanisms evolve from fee-for-service reimbursement to capitation or service line case rates the need for timely and accurate information processing increases.

Customer Service and Relationship Management

The notion of customer relationship management is highly relevant to health care information processing organizations. Customer relationship management is a step beyond "pleasing and delighting" and involves the availability of knowledge about the important elements of a customer's preferences and habits. In some retail businesses, customer service means knowing about a customer's purchases and preferences in style, size, fit, and timing. Ideally, patient management systems will have elements of the current medical record and problem list, prior utilization demographics, and plan information as well as information on preferences and service stipulations.

Complex, Adaptive Health Care Systems

Many integrated health care systems are complex organizations and may be described as "networked systems in continuous deliberations" (Pava, 1986). Health care delivery has been characterized as "organized complexity." Considering the conventional definition of system, a health care organization may actually appear to be a nonsystem, employing no centralized or uniform hierarchical management.

A fragmented and ineffective coordination of services, equipment, and facilities has existed in the past. The integration of a collaborating network of individually credentialed providers has been problematic. Regulatory concerns and a medicolegal liability labyrinth add to the complexity. Even clinical medicine seems to be fraught with shortcomings as "standards of care" based on peer-reviewed evidence seemingly apply to only a minority of clinical encounters. The complex interactions of multiple diseases, variable physiology, severity, functional status, economic status, psychology, and social roles create many uncertainties in the application and effectiveness of medical interventions.

"Complexity exists in an organized system when a large number of variables are functionally linked. . . . The system can become many possible states. The changing shape of the system obscures connections between structure and behavior" (Brunner & Brewer, 1977). Complex organizations in other industries are collections of semiautonomous agents that are interconnected informationally and that coordinate efforts automatically, acting as self-organizing collectives. These complex adaptive systems allow creativity, innovation, and emergent control. They are not subject to a centralized decision-dispersing body but are decentralized, to maximize their flexibility.

Complex, adaptive health care organizations have a survival advantage when information is integrated, workers are knowledge oriented, and control is distributed to self-organizing work groups.

Another characteristic of complex systems is that cause and effect relationships are obscured and may not be linear. Many of the results, or outcomes, in complex systems appear to be chaotic or random when in fact they are nonlinear and deterministic (exemplifying natural laws and having sufficient causes). Nonlinear systems theory develops "a powerful new tool set for understanding and manipulating processes, systems, organizations . . . [this tool set] allow[s] the visualization and management of nonlinear (apparent random and disordered) systems" (Sharp & Priesmeyer, 1995).

Emergent Control

Managing a complex system is a daunting task as prediction (relying on linear cause and effect), centralized control, and risk avoidance are not beneficial. Instead, leaders take an observational role and support and facilitate *emergent control*, in which solutions come forth from the fringes of the organization. Multiple options must be explored frequently, so risk taking and tolerance of failure are key characteristics. Frequently, coevolution and *coopetition* (cooperation and competition) are useful tactics because a bigger prize may exist if a larger market can be created. Spontaneous learning networks promote the generative relationships that are critical for collaboration and innovation. Managers of complex systems can foster this emergence through increased connectivity and information flow, designing an incentive to embrace collaboration and reduce territorialism.

Future health care organizations may be biological and social systems with inherent creativity and innovation that actualize information processing capability, demonstrating self-organization, adaptation, and self-regulation. These systems will have the characteristics of *open systems*, including constant exchange of ideas and exposure to new agents. *Closed systems*, in contrast, are mechanistic and predictable, with minimal exchange of information or interaction with the environment.

The Collaborative Information Processing Community

The social milieu in health care organizations must be addressed for successful information processing. The desired outcome of collaborative work should be a whole that is greater than the sum of its parts, yet this is difficult to attain.

What approaches stimulate collaboration? Sociotechnical systems theory specifies that the joint optimization of two critical subsystems of work, the technical and social, is necessary. This optimization enhances workers' creativity and innovation. The application known as self-directed work teams is one such approach to enhancing collaboration. It was discovered that organizations adopting this approach became self-regulating, interdependent, flexible, and able to handle uncertainty and complexity better. Formalized self-directed work teams have exemplified the characteristics of participative management, with multiskilled workers, minimum critical specifications, information channeled in a timely manner, variances managed at the point of care, ongoing redesign, and team performance measures.

In health care, this concept further evolved into the notion of patient-focused care, which employed teams of providers for patients with similar problems. Environments and workflow were, at times, radically redesigned along service delivery lines. Information delivery was recognized as a critical aspect of patient-focused care, with standardized vocabulary, integrated information, and point of care decision support that included clinical pathways, exception reporting, and event-driven triggers. Outcome analysis became possible and enabled performance accountability and the association of clinical with financial data.

Learning Networks

Another type of informal team or grouping of related workers is present in the health care information processing organization. In complex adaptive systems it has been noted that cohesive, formal teams are needed for day-to-day operations because they essentially replace typical management hierarchies. The other, more informal organization, sometimes referred to as the *shadow organization*, is frequently made up of spontaneous *learning networks* that have open dialogue and conflict and that are critical for handling strategic issues.

These learning networks can evolve to a more advanced state of collaboration, *communities of practice*. These communities are "self-organizing, regulating, informal networks of workers doing similar work, bound to one another through exposure to a common set of problems, embodying a store of knowledge in the common pursuit of solutions . . . driven by a mutual obligation to assist one another and having a sense of group accountability" (Manville & Foote, 1996b).

Diffusion of Innovation

Social communities of this nature serve an important role in the diffusion of innovation. Diffusion is "the process by which an innovation is communicated through certain channels over time among the members of a social system or organization" (Rogers, 1995). Innovations are new ideas associated with a degree of uncertainty, and diffusion of these new ideas is essentially social change. The diffusion process is driven by subjective evaluations of innovations that are acquired from opinion leaders and conveyed by informal interpersonal networks within communities of practice.

Frequently, an innovation undergoes reinvention by each community of practice. This is necessary for two reasons. First, the adopting organization may have certain unique requirements, and reinvention may result in a more appropriate match between a particular problem and the innovation. Second, the particular innovation must be aligned with the value system, mission, vision, and territories existing already in the organization. Communities of practice can foster helpful change and facilitate adoption of innovations through alignment of incentives in the existing social environment.

The Role of Technology

What is the role of technology in all of this? Rogers (1995) notes that technology encompasses "a design for instrumental (or computational) action that reduces uncertainty in potential cause and effect relationships." Health care decision support systems are designed with reducing uncertainty in mind, and such a system may be described as the "end to end process of gathering, structuring, manipulating, storing, accessing, presenting, and distributing actionable information" (Raden, 1995). This actionable information or knowledge may be obtained either immediately in response to a single operational transaction or more deliberately through analytical discovery in archived data.

Thus *health care decision support systems* seem to encompass two distinct processes: real-time proactive clinical decision support for single customer transactions and retrospective enterprise decision support systems for an analysis of historical trends. In reality, these two systems are closely linked. Analytical systems have the goal of deriving the *business rules* or *codes of action* that spell success and differentiate the enterprise from others. Operational systems ideally deploy the same business rules that have been derived by the analytical system. Of course the deployment of these rules, through computational approaches such as event-driven triggers and stored procedures, becomes substrate for the next iteration of the analytical system.

The distinction between *enterprise decision support* and *clinical decision support* completely dissipates when one is discussing the concept of the knowledge worker. Knowledge workers in health care represent the melding of the clerical function and the management function. Knowledge workers, as individuals within their communities of practice, derive and then deploy organizational knowledge during the course of delivering care.

Performance Improvement

Performance improvement in health care is essentially a process of discovery and creative activity carried out in an environment of scientific inquiry. Clinical knowledge workers transform data into information and information into knowledge.

Several key challenges confront them. Their lack of sufficient time to conduct studies and to research key questions emphasizes their need for efficient access to information. Another issue for knowledge workers is the capacity of the information systems: in order to measure longitudinal outcomes of care, large numbers of complex data elements must be stored and processed.

The ability of knowledge workers to communicate and disseminate information is vital to improvement activity. The fact that knowledge tends to be specialized makes it even more important that performance improvement analysts and clinical knowledge workers work in teams. Each individual has a great deal of specialized knowledge, but it is the team that creates the improvement in care.

Clinical knowledge workers must have access to information about processes of care to make decisions that will improve quality and better manage resources. Access to this information must be in real time to enable the improvement of care as it occurs.

Collaboration in an environment of inquiry across organizational boundaries encourages development of organizational knowledge. Knowledge workers can be most effective when they apply their knowledge interactively. A standardized clinical data model in performance improvement is also a critical success factor.

Decision support tools must empower the health care knowledge worker to study processes and outcomes of care in an efficient and standardized way to achieve improvement. It is beneficial, therefore, to empower clinical knowledge workers with information. Knowledge workers need acceptable response times and ease of access as they seek information. Clinical workstations that have direct query capabilities and that allow knowledge workers to review integrated information across the continuum of care facilitate those workers' understandings of clinical processes.

Clinical knowledge workers improve quality by recognizing and ultimately eliminating process variation through appropriate information at the point of care. Enhanced information provided to the knowledge worker can improve effectiveness and efficiency and ultimately create value. Non-value-added activities of the knowledge worker are eliminated as duplication and redundancy are minimized. Information technology at the point of care fosters the creation of a knowledge community and supports the empowered knowledge workers in their journey of discovery.

Data Mining and Discovery

Data mining is the process of discovering meaningful associations, patterns, and trends by scrutinizing large amounts of data stored in data warehouses with various pattern recognition, statistical, and visualization techniques. To a limited extent, data mining technologies can be applied to operational data for the same discovery purposes.

As noted previously, health care information processing organizations require analytical decision support capabilities when using cumulative historical data to uncover trends, patterns, and business rules, and they require operational decision support capabilities when using individual real-time data to deploy rules or evidence. Data mining facilitates analysis and the process of uncovering historical trends, patterns, and associations. These technologies support knowledge workers in their quest to identify innovations and improve the performance of health care delivery processes.

Data mining is complementary to data warehousing and requires a carefully planned information processing architecture, data model, and data warehouse to be successful (see Chapter Four). A data mining system has two major considerations: (1) the model, which is usually based on prior knowledge and behavior under conditions of certainty, and (2) the computational forecast or prediction under conditions of uncertainty. Several technologies and models are used in data mining:

- Case-based reasoning, a methodology that classifies new cases based on their similarity to previous known cases

- Data visualization, a process of using graphical and visually enhanced methods to accent trends or patterns

- Fuzzy logic, a technique to categorize items by clustering relevant attributes and estimating closeness of fit

- Knowledge discovery, the use of statistical methods, such as regression, to determine significance of correlation

- Neural networks, models that forecast results based on prior training set through a computational system, with predetermined weights applied to specific attributes

- Decision trees, models that result from using rules in sequence to direct an algorithm classification scheme

- Genetic algorithms, procedures that categorize the evolution-ary nature of various combinations of multiple variables and quantify the results to assess the emergence of ecologically optimal solutions

Conclusion

The health care information processing organization is a knowl-edge-driven enterprise, fully employing the collective knowledge of its workers. The social environment in such organizations can be described as a complex, adaptive system that has the attributes of diversity, formal and informal interaction, risk taking, decentral-ization, and emergent control. Social communities of practice, made up of health care workers sharing a common vision, sponta-neously arise to meet customers' and patients' custom needs and desires. This promotes an atmosphere of creativity, discovery, and innovation that fosters the trajectory of change required for health care delivery systems to compete in the twenty-first century.

Chapter Four

The Health Care Information Processing Environment

The Technical Infrastructure

Roy E. Gilbreath

The information processing organization must support the clinical knowledge worker with new kinds of interaction and transfer of knowledge. This chapter describes this supportive information processing architecture, the communities it serves, its components (data warehouses, operational data stores, and data marts), and the components' structure, function, enablers, and tools. It also discusses an integrated approach to the clinical workstation, so that it uses both on-line transaction processing and on-line analytic processing applications in health care delivery.

The last chapter outlined the conceptual model for the health care information processing organization and the social environment needed to support a successful knowledge-based enterprise. Cultivating knowledge by supporting knowledge workers in collaborative behaviors is the key for success. Knowledge workers, by necessity, interact at the critical juncture in the operational process (the transactions with customers) but must be supported in these transactions by the knowledge of the whole enterprise. No longer can a knowledge worker be regarded as a backroom analyst, never interacting at the point of service. These workers and the enterprise knowledge base must interact in real time at the customer interface.

The information delivery system must support these kinds of interactions through two key mechanisms: the first facilitates unimpeded information flow between knowledge workers; the second offers contextual decision support, which may be simple historical fact, as in results reporting, or a synthesis of multiple existing facts, as in an expert system.

Both of these mechanisms serve to create knowledge pull; they cue the knowledge worker during patient transactions for the purpose of influencing these transactions in a positive way. Remember that not all transactions will have a predefined organizational approach. In fact, only a minority of transactions may be manageable solely through existing guidelines. The majority are likely to reflect an underlying complexity owing to such factors as comorbidities; social, psychological, or financial constraints; patient preferences; physiological variation; medical evidence variation (more than one standard of care); and practice variation (as a result of regional or institutional issues).

In these situations of uncertainty and nonuniform agreement, emergent control will evolve if a free flow of information among agents occurs. Variations from guidelines are likely to be handled successfully at the point of service by knowledge workers who are guided by fundamentals (mission, vision, general standards of care) and who demonstrate creativity and innovation in a collaborative solution.

Therefore, knowledge workers are semiautonomous agents in contact with patients at key junctures in service delivery and must be supported both for *known standard operations* (deploying organizational rules) and for *analysis or synthesis of unknown processes* (deriving new rules in uncharted or changing clinical terrain). We cannot expect knowledge workers to use separate systems (with separate workstations) to accomplish different approaches. Their entree to the enterprise knowledge store should be uniform and transparent. Modern standards for vocabulary, middleware, security, and user access can enable this vision.

Information Processing Architecture

The information processing architecture that supports this environment has specific constructs that are not contained in most legacy systems, that is, existing older computerized systems. These legacy systems have typically evolved in increments, with best-of-breed applications interfacing with point-to-point, often proprietary programs. Often, there is no standardization between systems, so information derived from one area of the enterprise might appear to be completely different from the same fact derived from another area.

Why do discrepancies occur? Differences in vocabulary, meaning, methodology, subject population, and merged external data may all contribute. It is very expensive to correct these problems, as navigating through the spider web maze and attempting to standardize at the various points of service is next to impossible. Furthermore, these legacy architectures demonstrate lack of flexibility when the organization is changing to a new standard, because of the many point-to-point proprietary interfaces that must be simultaneously reengineered and retrofitted.

As health care information systems grew and developed, information managers attempted to resolve these issues by implementing *central data repositories*. The central repository model deployed a central database management system (frequently proprietary) on a single computer in a central location. It was a hub-and-spoke system, and it required many point-to-point proprietary interfaces. Health Level 7 (HL7) middleware was an attempt to ease the resulting application–repository interface burden but addressed only data format standards.

Problems became apparent when these systems were operationalized. As long as transaction demands were at a minimum, processing time was acceptable. Once transaction data traffic and archived data became significant, unacceptable delays occurred, especially when analytical decision support queries were processed simultaneously with operations.

Entity Relationship Model

Another problem became apparent with the entity relationship model and relational database management system (RDBMS). This type of data modeling and the resultant structure and query methodologies were optimized for rapid, high-performance transaction processing. The basic functions of an RDBMS were to update certain data fields of interest and delete redundant information. By necessity, the relational database had to eliminate any redundancy, a process known as normalization. Otherwise, multiple tables and fields required simultaneous update and deletion procedures whenever a change was noted, greatly increasing processing time and decreasing system performance. So relational database technology was optimized for real-time on-line transaction processing (OLTP) and could do an exemplary job at this, but it placed a significant restriction on the data model by requiring it to eliminate any redundancy. Ultimately, it became apparent that relational database systems had difficulty accessing stored data and getting these data out. A structured query language (SQL) was developed in an attempt to standardize database query methodology and allow cross-querying between relational database management systems. Soon, SQL was touted as the ultimate query language for decision support on archived RDBMS. Ironically, SQL never offered much support for basic decision support queries concerning such issues as comparisons, slowly changing dimensions, or questions involving temporal dimensions.

In addition, SQL and the entity relationship model, which was two-dimensional and accompanied by a labyrinth of interrelated tables, were not easy for users, analysts, or knowledge workers to navigate. Organizations began delegating decision support to the backroom analysts who could speak SQL and understood the entity relationship diagram, which typically spanned an entire office wall (Figure 4.1).

Furthermore, it became apparent that an RDBMS using SQL could answer who, what, when, where, and how, but had difficulty

Figure 4.1. OLTP Schema: Entity Relationship Model.

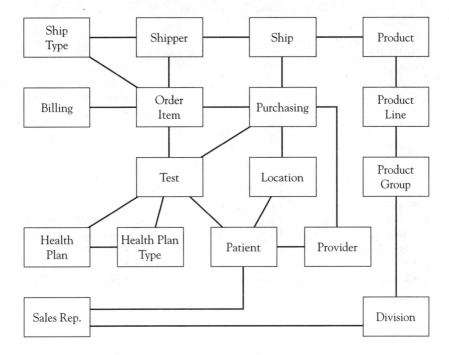

in illuminating why, mainly because of its limited capabilities to make comparisons (Kimball, 1996).

Something more was needed, and in the mid 1980s, Ralph Kimball began pointing out the difficulties with employing relational technology for decision support. As a result, dimensional modeling, specifically designed for decision support, evolved. Characteristically, redundancy was deliberately introduced in certain dimensions (a process known as denormalization), and this model became known as the *star join schema* (Figure 4.2). Performance on existing RDBMSs was still a problem; however, the use of aggregate summaries and other technological features, such as bit-mapped indexing, enabled acceptable performance on very large databases, or *data warehouses*, in the terabyte range.

Figure 4.2. Dimensional Data Warehouse (DDW):
Star Join Schema.

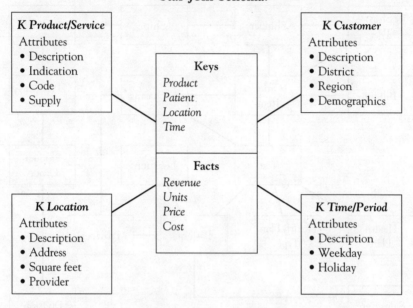

Information Processing Architecture

Introduced as the preferred architecture for decision support systems, the data warehouse concept, employing dimensional modeling, was advanced by William Inmon (1993) in the late 1980s. Successful decision support systems required that the data warehouse employ a physical (hardware) platform and logical (data model) platform separate from the operational system. It soon became apparent that once an operational, transaction-driven system was "liberated from the need to archive past historical data," it could perform better (Inmon, 1993). Only current data needed to be housed on the OLTP system and then snapshots of these data could be transferred to the data warehouse. Relieved of historical data, the operational system showed greatly improved performance times. Data transformation, storage, query, and presentation were now the problem of the data warehouse administrator. Eventually, developers created another component known as the *operational data store*, an operational system that integrated critical information across multiple legacy systems. The operational data store had a defined time horizon and was distinct from the data warehouse (Inmon, Imhoff, & Battas, 1995) (Figure 4.3).

Health care organizations must continue to beware of operational data repositories that have an unlimited archive. They typically experience serious performance problems, and although the rationale that "advances in hardware technology" will solve these problems is frequently mentioned, other industries have found that such advances have not solved the problems that arise when knowledge workers attempt to execute decision support queries on an operational system.

In summary, current information processing architecture features the dual constructs of the data warehouse and operational data store, which serve distinct purposes and functions:

- The data warehouse has the purpose of supporting analytical workers in long-term decision making, with the goal of deriving enterprise business and clinical rules.

Figure 4.3. Characteristics of Operational Data Stores and Data Warehouses.

Operational Data Store	Data Warehouse
Is volatile	Is nonvolatile
Supports clinicians	Supports management
Has a short time horizon	Has an extended time horizon
Supports immediate decisions	Supports long-term decisions
Contains homogeneous data	Contains heterogeneous data
Offers high performance	Performance relaxed
Uses relational modeling	Uses multidimensional modeling
Uses SQL	Uses multidimensional analysis
Deploys business rules	Derives business rules
Manages outcomes	Analyzes outcomes

- The operational data store has the purpose of supporting operational workers in immediate or short-term decision making, with the goal of deploying the enterprise business and clinical rules.

- The data warehouse has the function of exploiting the data through analysis, identification of trends (*trending*); summarization, or aggregation (*rolling up*); and separation (*drilling down* from less detailed to more detailed data), and it specializes in supporting retrospective, tactical, and strategic reporting.

- The operational data store has the function of capturing the data accurately through standardization, correction, discrepancy resolution, and process automation, and it offers real-time operational control, with event-driven triggers and stored procedures.

What are the differences in the design of the two constructs? The data warehouse and operational data store have completely different models, design, hardware, and software requirements, as defined by the distinct functional expectations.

The data warehouse is created from time-stamped, granular operational data, indexed into a metadata table of contents, and in many cases aggregated and summarized into categories such as regions, periods, and types, as defined by business necessity.

The process of converting operational time-stamped data to the data warehouse format is called data transformation. This is no small task and is generally noted by experts to be the most challenging aspect of data warehouse implementation.

The transformation process would not be that difficult if all the important terms used by the enterprise were embodied in a standardized vocabulary. However, in reality, vocabulary is varied and needs to be standardized. A single clinical finding, for example, may be described by one of several medical terms.

Figure 4.4 is a schematic portrayal of the information processing architecture. As we have been discussing, there are two distinct

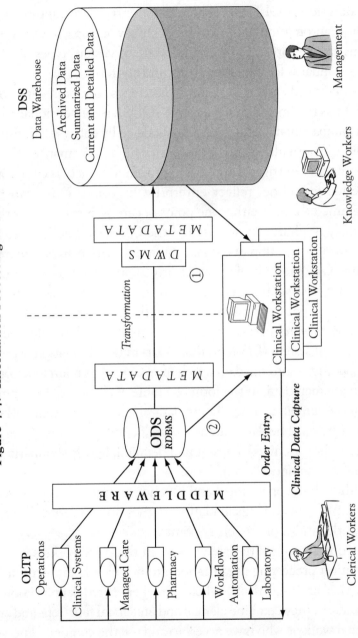

Figure 4.4. Information Processing Architecture.

DSS
Data Warehouse

Archived Data
Summarized Data
Current and Detailed Data

Management

Knowledge Workers

METADATA

DWMS

①

Transformation

METADATA

ODS
RDBMS

②

Clinical Workstation
Clinical Workstation
Clinical Workstation

Clinical Data Capture

Order Entry

MIDDLEWARE

OLTP
Operations

Clinical Systems

Managed Care

Pharmacy

Workflow
Automation

Laboratory

Clerical Workers

① Parameters, reminders, data mining, routine results, archived CPR   ② Alerts, triggers, urgent results, guidelines, operational CPR environments: the operational data store and the data warehouse, also known as the decision support system (DSS). Operations' main function is OLTP, to enable order entry, data capture, and workflow automation with extreme accuracy and speed. Disparate systems can be integrated by middleware of various types, which creates standards for data formatting and content.

As described earlier, the central data repository, possessing current data, is the operational data store (ODS), a conventional relational database management system, modeled by entity relationship techniques, normalized and optimized for high performance.

Event-driven triggers and stored procedures, such as cues from a practice guideline, reflect enterprise knowledge and can be programmed through either the point of care systems (such as the laboratory or pharmacy systems) or the ODS, especially if cross-application integration of data is required to derive an automated response. One example of an event-driven procedure is examining laboratory data such as serum creatinine to effect a response in the form of a patient's pharmaceutical dosing (Figure 4.5).

The data warehouse environment consists of a data warehouse management system (DWMS) that assists in transformation of data from operations into the data warehouse. One of its main functions is to create metadata, in the form of a table of contents, describing the various *attributes* of warehouse data such as source, summaries, and definitions. The data warehouse itself contains several types of data including archived, current and detailed, lightly summarized, and highly summarized data.

Although the operational and warehouse environments possess separate physical and logical platforms, they are not served by separate workstations or user entry points.

In contrast to health care workers in the past, workers in the information processing organization are not clearly differentiated into clerical and analytical. As Peter Drucker (1985) defined knowledge workers, they combine clerical and analytical functions and are relational workers who have access to and use the corporate knowl-

Figure 4.5. Information Processing as a Decision-Making Tool.

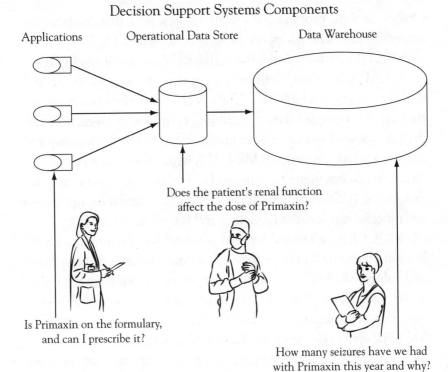

Decision Support Systems Components

Applications   Operational Data Store   Data Warehouse

Does the patient's renal function
affect the dose of Primaxin?

Is Primaxin on the formulary,
and can I prescribe it?

How many seizures have we had
with Primaxin this year and why?

edge base to make better operational decisions, usually in real time. Knowledge workers frequently require enterprise knowledge to make operational real-time decisions. They understand that simple transactions should be fast and that trending may take longer.

Data marts describe the departmental subsets of the enterprise data warehouse, such as the data areas for cardiovascular medicine, oncology, or orthopedics. An enterprise will have multiple data marts supporting its functional areas. Knowledge workers may interact with data marts to discover enterprise business and clinical rules, and they use various tools for querying, reporting, and online analytic processing (OLAP).

Querying, Reporting, and OLAP

On-line analytic processing is a relatively new term that describes the activities of a decision support, or analytical, system. OLAP contrasts with OLTP, which describes the activities of an operational system.

OLAP, which is rapidly replacing the previous querying and reporting tools available to OLTP systems, describes two methods that analyze complex data by enabling comparison, trend analysis, drill down, and roll up. These methods are (1) multidimensional on-line analytic processing (MOLAP), which uses proprietary *cubed* database management systems, and (2) relational on-line analytic processing (ROLAP), which uses relational databases, optimized with special star schema modeling and bit-mapped indexing.

MOLAP is best suited for analyses in which the dimensions are both unchanging and bounded with a limited number of attributes and values. MOLAP is limited by the size of the database but is easier to maintain and update and usually performs faster because of the data reaggregation and summarization required. Typically, MOLAP systems support smaller departmental data marts.

ROLAP systems can support larger, detailed data marts or warehouses but are difficult to update and typically are not as fast as MOLAP systems because aggregates are calculated "on the fly." ROLAP systems are more flexible and open to change and are applicable when dimensions are fluid and changing. Exploration of the data is facilitated on the ROLAP engines because of the access to detailed data, but ROLAP requires much more skill and time on the part of the analyst.

Three types of analysts use the OLAP engines: *tourists, farmers,* and *explorers* (Inmon, Imhoff, & Sousa, 1998). Tourists prefer a *dashboard* of highly relevant, readily accessible, summary information. They rarely go beyond the initial information, usually delegating detailed investigation to someone else. Farmers are more inquisitive and are willing to work harder and longer to get results, but still prefer a high return on the time invested in the analysis.

Farmers are satisfied most of the time by preformatted queries with standard drill-down, roll-up, comparison, and trending detail. Explorers insist on ad hoc query capability (that is, the means of formatting queries for their specific needs of the moment) and rely heavily on iteration, or repetition of queries based on the results of the former query. Explorers will devote many hours to the investigation of a hunch and will not be deterred by the failure of an analysis to show significance. They love the hunt of an investigation and will be satisfied if they only occasionally have success. Both explorers and farmers frequently say, "Show me what I say I want, then I will tell you what I really want."

Data Modeling

The dimensional data modeling method, through standardization of definitions and the creation of uniform conforming dimensions, serves to integrate data in the warehouse, thus enabling summary and comparison. Most existing health care delivery systems have multiple best-of-breed operational applications. Order entry, results reporting, laboratory records, radiology records, medical records, administrative records, and financial records may all be on separate systems, all requiring a certain amount of redundant data entry and each with its own data element definitions, processes, storage, and interpretation algorithms. In this situation the enterprise data is nonintegrated.

One of the primary goals and benefits of the information processing architecture is integration of data, and in most environments this necessitates standardization of vocabularies and processes. These activities of standardization, which are primarily social tasks, become the most daunting and time consuming activities in an information processing architecture implementation and utilization initiative. This initiative cannot succeed without standardization of vocabulary and processes (moreover, this standardization is valuable to the enterprise apart from the initiative).

Standardization of definitions and meanings is critical to the dimensional data modeling process, because of the requirements for uniform conforming dimensions across the enterprise. Earlier we discussed the distinct data modeling technique used by the data warehouse and known as dimensional modeling (Figure 4.2) and pointed out that the deliberate introduction of redundancy in the attributes, which describe the characteristics of the dimensions, makes for easier and more complete queries but does add the complication of diminished performance in terms of speed. However, accuracy of the results may be enhanced in the dimensional model, and this is attributed to the technical differences in the ways the relational model (Figure 4.1) and the dimensional model are queried.

The star join schema of the dimensional model is built around a given subject domain, or dimension, such as a service line, type of patient, function, or discipline. Many different domain-specific star join schemas can be combined in an enterprise model as long as each schema has conforming dimensional attributes, or the same possible set of values for similarly described dimensions. A star join schema is composed of a centralized table of facts (*fact table*) attached to multiple tables of attributes (*dimension tables*). The facts in a given domain are data that are numeric, additive, and continually valued and that can be summarized in some way. The number of admissions or positive test results are good numeric facts, for example.

Attributes in the dimensional table describe the domain under study (for example, they are adjectives describing a noun) and are typically textual and discretely and uniquely valued. The attributes are important because they become the source of constraints and, in spreadsheet parlance, the row headers. Examples of attributes are date, size, diagnosis, and procedure code.

A chief characteristic of the dimensional model is that the same attributes may be repeated in several dimensional tables, which is the process known as denormalization, as described previously. Remember, one aspect of query performance is speed, and repeating attributes greatly increases the updating required in multiple seek and replace tasks and therefore affects performance adversely for an RDBMS supporting OLTP. Speed of processing is critically important in real-time, transaction-based operational systems, and a decline in this area can have negative impacts on production and patient care efficiency. The analytical environment does not require quite the same degree of speed, as most users intuitively understand that a trending query, which analyzes lots of data over time, may take several seconds, whereas simple updates in transaction processing should occur almost immediately, in a subsecond response. Therefore, it is expected that the operational environment will be speed performance sensitive and the analytical environment speed performance relaxed.

Another aspect of query performance is quality, completeness, and accuracy. In this area, the dimensional model clearly has an advantage, by virtue of its attribute redundancy and ability to aggregate or summarize relevant facts. Therefore, the trade-off is between speed and precision. Relational models optimize for speed; dimensional models optimize for accuracy, completeness, and interpretability.

A further significant aspect of the dimensional model is the way the central fact table is related to the surrounding dimensional tables. In the generic star join schema, the keys in the central fact table are dimensional table subjects (in Figure 4.2, for example, they are product, location, customer, and time). Other subjects relevant to health care that might be keys are health plan, health status, and outcomes (Figure 4.2).

In database modeling, both relational and dimensional, these relationships between tables are critical. As we have noted, in the entity relationship model the relationships between tables become quite convoluted and, in a complex system, virtually uninterpretable to even an educated user (Figure 4.1). The dimensional model, however, remains to a large degree understandable, which definitely promotes the end user's ability to do ad hoc, or exploratory, queries, enabling knowledge discovery by workers close to the customer. Indeed, clinical knowledge workers have a role not only as users of the corporate knowledge base but as discoverers. Most of them, being detectives already as they care for patients, feel quite comfortable in this role.

Metadata

Compiled into a table of contents, metadata form one of the most important aspects of the information processing architecture. Metadata make possible the directory for the data in the data warehouse and data marts but are equally important in describing the operational data store and the source applications systems. They must be carefully constructed during the data modeling and transformation phases. They play a large role in the determination of data quality, as they include information about the data, its sources, and its transformation. Frequently, applications data are not standardized and must be integrated, altered, and classified before their transformation into the data warehouse. These *technical* metadata track the rules by which the data elements are integrated into the warehouse.

In contrast, *business* (clinical) metadata are what data analysts use when touring, farming, or exploring the data warehouse. Present metadata systems are rich in business (or clinical) descriptors, allowing natural language interpretation rather than obscure coding. Business metadata systems should always be available on-line and able to be referenced in real time, assisting the analyst in query formulation.

Conclusion

Information technology supports and empowers clinical knowledge workers in their journeys of discovery. The health care information processing architecture is the technical infrastructure that supports both the operational and analytical environments. It has been established that effective operational and analysis functions require separate data models, technology platforms, and architectural constructs. The operational environment consists of legacy systems; point of care, or departmental, applications; and the operational data store. The analysis environment consists of the data warehouse.

The function of the operational system is to optimize high accuracy and speed in the transactions that deliver care to the customer. The function of the analytical system is data storage, analysis, and presentation. Knowledge workers should be able to derive the enterprise business and clinical rules through the analytical system. Knowledge workers can then deploy those same business and clinical rules with the help of the operational system, through an integrated clinical workstation.

This information processing architecture supports the health care information processing organization in performance improvement, change management, accountability, and strategic management, making possible a competitive health care delivery enterprise.

Chapter Five

Provider-Sponsored Coordinated Care Organizations

Designing Systems for Patient-Centered Care

Roy E. Gilbreath

Traditional fee-for-service cottage industry
medicine has given way to insurer-sponsored
managed care delivery systems, which typically use
oversight methodologies for obtaining cost
efficiencies. Proponents of continuous quality
improvement understand that *oversight and
inspection* is not ideal and advocate *process
innovation* and *quality by design* instead. Provider-
sponsored coordinated care organizations (PCCOs)
have the potential to develop mechanisms of
health care delivery based on collaboration across
the continuum, process innovation, and design of
systems that provide superior outcomes and
efficient delivery of services. This chapter explains
how the management of information will play a
pivotal role in the ability of these health care
organizations to meet purchasers', payers', and
patients' demands.

"Provider-Sponsored Coordinated Care Organizations: Designing Systems for Patient-
Centered Care" is reprinted with permission from *Healthcare Information Management*,
Fall 1996, *10* (3). ©Healthcare Information and Management Systems Society and
Jossey-Bass Inc., Publishers.

Managed care entities have made great strides in obtaining cost efficiencies in health care delivery while maintaining quality and reasonable patient satisfaction. It is suspected by many that this progress has been obtained primarily by aligning providers' incentives and creating systems of oversight, such as traditional utilization review.

Providers have responded by consolidating into functionally integrated groups and, in addition, have begun to create their own programs in quality, outcomes, and resource management. Payers are allowing these medical groups to provide these services and in some cases reimbursing them, especially if savings are generated from successful utilization management.

More recently, payers have become very interested in contracting with provider-owned, -directed, and -driven networks. These may encompass traditional group practices with economically integrated physician providers or independent providers organized in an independent practice association (IPA). One advantage of an IPA in this setting is broader market coverage and a more appealing fit of members to providers. In certain progressive markets, providers have organized systems of *coordinated care* that strive for high-quality, cost-efficient health care delivery using many creative and innovative programs for prevention, access to care, patient compliance, guidelines adherence, and resource management.

Information systems must support workflow automation and deployment of decision-making tools at the point of care. Standardization of data vocabulary and definitions will be required for effective analysis and management of outcomes. An appropriately planned and designed informational processing architecture with technical standards delineation is an important early consideration. Issues of compatibility, sharing of data, connectivity, and integration can be addressed judiciously if the technical architecture and standards requirements have been outlined beforehand.

Provider organizations will increasingly be responsible for and take on the full scope of quality, resource, and outcomes management; claims processing, contract, and funds management; provider services, credentialing, network, and capacity management; and, more importantly, member services, which will progressively include more care coordination services that ensure access to care and satisfaction.

Information systems and associated technology must evolve with these new delivery systems. This is a significant departure from the traditional health care informatics focus on institutional care. Instead, PCCOs will serve predominantly ambulatory patients with a focus on prevention of illness and improvement of the health status of the regional community served. It can be expected that a heavy emphasis on clinical improvement, to obtain superior medical and service outcomes, will be the focus of these new organizations.

The information system requirements to support these PCCOs are extensive and complex. The marketplace can be characterized as multiple vendor offerings on various platforms, often with overlapping functionality.

Organizations embracing coordinated care need a formalized approach to systems evaluation and selection. They need to use a structured methodology that involves as many stakeholders as possible to obtain both valuable input and knowledge worker ownership, which will be important for the future implementation.

Initially organizations should make an inventory of information requirements, both internal and external. They should delineate and standardize data elements and their definitions, ideally in a consensus-driven process.

Rather than choosing off-the-shelf vendor applications, they should first delineate an information processing architecture, encompassing appropriate standards for software, operating systems, and hardware. Usually, the *managed care information system*, for claims processing, funds management, and utilization management, is the first system to be evaluated. In time, practice management systems, clinical documentation systems, point-of-care applications addressing workflow, and clinical decision support systems will be evaluated. The longitudinal electronic health record will evolve from these systems and others. Additional systems to consider are severity adjustment applications and enterprise communications. It is best to evaluate each of these systems through the formal approach called the *systems development life cycle* (SDLC), using requests for proposal (RFPs) for vendor evaluation and selection. In this way, the user controls the process and maximizes the possibility of successful requirements delineation, vendor evaluation and selection, and implementation.

Evolution to Coordinated Care

Traditional health care delivery was typically a fragmented, informal, and uncoordinated cottage industry, centered on providers. Fee-for-service medicine predominated and was characterized by considerable variation in process, quality, and outcomes, as well as unconstrained profit maximization by entrepreneurial providers and institutions.

Managed care has been a response to employer demands for accountable health plans, which were successfully constructed by the HMO industry. These payers attained cost efficiencies while maintaining equal or better quality care by using the oversight model, which involves inspection and policing of decisions that have a high impact on costs. The managed care environment has become, in many ways, payer centered.

Coordinated care implies provider sponsorship and looks to innovative, reengineered processes that are centered on patients. This has even greater potential for attaining high-quality, improved outcomes and better cost efficiencies because it requires fundamental process redesign. Even well-established payers realize that gains from the oversight model are limited, and they too embrace *coordinated care* and *partnerships* with willing provider organizations.

The goal of a PCCO is to increase the value of health care delivery, according to the value equation (see Figure 1.1). Quality relates to effectiveness, or *doing the right thing*. Cost relates to efficiency, or *doing it right*.

A coordinated care organization may be conceived of as a *tiered delivery system*. The ultimate goal of a coordinated care system is to provide care to the patient at the right time, in the right place, in the right degree to attain favorable outcomes, high access and satisfaction, and optimum functional status while being cost efficient. The coordinated care organization does not merely respond to patient demands but also preempts health issues and advocates for healthy lifestyle changes and proactive disease management while ensuring access to appropriate care. Preventing avoidable medical events and costs and improving the health status of the community of patients served are integral strategies of coordinated care organizations.

Many popular movements are encompassed in the tiers of care of a coordinated care organization. Among them are self-care programs, demand management, disease state management, case management, pharmaceutical care, geriatric care management, telephone triage, and integrated scheduling. Patients are appropriately routed to midlevel providers, ancillary services, primary care physicians, and specialists as well as hospital, emergency, or tertiary institutional services.

Demand management has primarily a disease prevention focus. The major elements of patient satisfaction, education, and access to care are pivotal to the success of these programs. Demand management does not merely address ways of alleviating the demands patients may put on a delivery system but also advocates for preemptive action to reduce requirements for future medical interventions.

Disease state management addresses disease manifestations and has typically focused on high-cost and high-morbidity conditions, such as diabetes and asthma. The pharmaceutical industry, fearing that restrictive drug formularies would result in HMO *lockout*, has retooled its strategies around disease state management. The resulting protocols, guidelines, and pathways certainly can assist providers in appropriate decision making. Disease state management has a preventive focus and a focus on common scenarios related to serious illness such as diabetes with vasculopathy result-ing from poorly controlled glucose, exemplified in glycohemoglo-bin monitoring.

Case management typically involves a catastrophic condition such as HIV, congestive heart failure, or cancer. Hospice care can be considered case management at the end of life. In many cases, payers have created case management programs to hedge against catastrophic costs.

Resource management employs optimum scheduling and resource planning and ensures access to care through facilitation and matching of patient needs and expectations with deliverable services.

Data Demands: External and Internal

PCCOs can expect to be required to produce the same reports as any other *accountable health plans*. There are many regulatory requirements emanating from organizations such as the National Committee for Quality Assurance (NCQA), the Joint Commis-sion on Accreditation of Healthcare Organizations, the Health Care Financing Administration, and state agencies. In addition, to compete in managed care environments, organizations are fre-quently required to undertake routine profiling of both the providers and the plan and comparison benchmarking with national clinical repositories.

In particular it is already commonplace for purchasers to require NCQA certification. Virtually every private organization is approaching the Health Plan Employer Data and Information Set (HEDIS) reporting with great attention. The HEDIS parameters primarily address quality of care (prevention, disease management), member access and satisfaction, membership utilization (hospital services, procedures), financial performance, and health plan man-agement. PCCOs may be required by their insurance partners to supply much of the information required in HEDIS reporting for eventual NCQA certification.

Internal reporting demands are generally focused around continuous quality improvement (CQI). Outcomes reporting, analysis, and management are extremely important. Ideally, interim process measures will be linked to outcomes to attain *clinical practice improvement* and linked to costs to enable *activity-based costing and management*. The result should be ongoing resource efficiency and outcomes improvement.

Provider profiling makes possible calibration of the organization to the marketplace. Provider *report cards* have operational value because they are frequently made the basis for incentive compensation. Balanced report cards assessing satisfaction, access to care, functional status, outcomes, and utilization are critical. *Profiling* of departments and institutions is of tactical value for internal CQI efforts. These measurements are frequently the basis for determining provider group performance and also a source for calculating incentive compensation. Organizational *dashboards* are of strategic value as defined outlines of success factors and processes. These three types of profiles are extremely important because they enable the organization to calibrate its services to external market demands.

Competitiveness in any product or service industry will rely on one of two strategies. One is differentiation, which in health care is based on quality issues such as medical outcomes, functional status, or service matters, such as satisfaction and access to care. Another strategy is price leadership. Ultimately, however, price must accurately reflect the cost of delivery of services, a historically difficult task in health care. Price leadership is highly dependent on process efficiency but is also related to quality concerns, as reductions in health care rework, quality waste, and delays in providing appropriate care are critical determinants for costs.

In the coordinated care organization, information systems must support the collection, analysis, reporting, and management of outcomes, including medical, service, and cost outcomes. The advantages of PCCOs are built around effective network management (matching of members to providers) and the coordination of services as well as medical management focusing on attainment of optimal medical, service, and cost outcomes. The obstacles to outcomes management have traditionally been multiple, unintegrated, departmentalized databases; nonstandardized vocabulary and definitions; lack of credibility and validity in available data; lack of flexibility to meet changing demands; and costly, inefficient data analysis.

Outcomes management programs ultimately must facilitate clinical practice improvement. Such interventions are successful when they are applied incrementally, use standard data definitions and vocabularies, ensure confidentiality and security, guarantee data validity and accurate severity of illness adjustment, support an educational not a punitive emphasis toward knowledge workers, and focus on processes linked to outcomes and cost.

Decision Support Systems

The notion of information processing in support of outcomes management is embodied in the term *decision support systems*. Decision support systems have two distinct components: enterprise decision support, focusing on the retrospective, analytical processing of data, and clinical decision support, focusing on prospective, real-time, transaction processing interventions.

Enterprise decision support systems use historical data for the purposes of analysis and reporting. Typically, the goal is to assess effectiveness (Are we doing the right thing?) and efficiency (Are we doing it right?). The system attempts to derive business and clinical rules for the enterprise and to serve as an enabler of quality by inspection. Enterprise decision support systems use data warehouse and on-line analytical processing (OLAP) technologies to achieve their goals.

Clinical decision support systems use current data for proactive interventions in the form of alerts, reminders, guidelines, pathways, and parameters. The effort is to *foolproof* clinical and business processes. These systems strive to *do it right the first time, every time*.

Functioning at the point of service, they attempt to deploy business and clinical rules derived from either national standards of care or data analysis of enterprise decision support systems. Ultimately, clinical decision support systems enable quality by design.

A PCCO requires an information processing architecture that supports outcomes management, facilitates reporting, enables quality improvement and resource management, and supports the electronic global or longitudinal health record over a regional area with multiple linked and distributed offices, agencies, institutions, payers, and purchasers. These information systems must support collecting and reporting of retrospective information and also the work of prospective management and improvement. This requires technical architecture that separates operational or transaction processing from analytical processing, physically and logically.

Ralph Kimball (1996), a pioneer in data warehousing and decision support systems (as discussed in Chapter Four), has stated that "decision support data management systems are invariably multidimensional."

Multidimensional databases are an outgrowth of executive information systems. They are optimized for flexibility of output and effective data presentation. The dimensions are intuitive business constructs, such as customer, provider, service, and location. Multidimensional analysis is enabled by various end-user tool sets available in the marketplace. They support OLAP and trend analysis with such techniques as pivot tables (analyzing from different perspectives), rolling up (aggregating), drilling down (separating), and performing built-in calculations. Today, common spreadsheet functionality encompasses many of these abilities. Indeed, multidimensional analysis blends many traditional relational database and common spreadsheet features.

The appropriate architecture to support information processing that will in turn support a coordinated care organization consists of two components, as outlined in Chapter Four: the *data warehouse*, which supports analytical workers and management in their long term decision making, and the *operational data store*, which supports transaction workers (clinicians) for immediate short-term decision making.

The data warehouse is defined (Inmon, 1993) as a "subject oriented, integrated, non-volatile, time variant collection of data in support of management decisions." In health care the *subjects* of the data warehouse are product or service lines, patient groups, diseases, or disease groupings. *Integrated* data are standardized, with unambiguous and accepted data definitions. Data warehouse data are *nonvolatile* because they are unchanging. They are *time variant* because each element has been stamped as recorded at a particular moment in time. The data in the data warehouse are modeled for optimum analysis and presentation and are thus fundamentally different from operational data. In addition, the appropriate architecture requires physical and logical separation of operational and data warehouse platforms. The data warehouse is made up of integrated enterprise data that is separate from operational data. Operational data is transformed into warehouse data through a process of cleansing, scrubbing, and partitioning, which can be accomplished by several commercial software packages.

During transformation, the creation of a metadata directory is required. This is a directory to the contents and location of data throughout the enterprise, and it contains facts about data modeling and structure, source and origin, and transformation. Ultimately, the goal of data analysis in the data warehouse is to allow the trending of key subject areas, to support data analysis over the long term, and to derive the enterprise business or clinical rules that distinguish the enterprise from its competitors.

There are many commercial products available that support various functions within the data warehouse, including multidimensional database management systems, analysis and presentation systems, and transformation and metadata management systems. Data warehouses are ideally implemented incrementally, starting with an inexpensive pilot of modest proportions with clear-cut expected benefits. The project should use iterative prototyping and constant system adjustment to meet the needs of data analysts.

The steps are as follows: create the data model (multidimensional); define the system of record, or the definitive source of operational data; design the warehouse; transform the data; populate the warehouse; and complete the feedback from the data analyst to the data warehouse architects.

The other major component of information processing architecture is the operational data store (ODS). The ODS is subject oriented, integrated, and volatile and reflects a current or near current collection of data in support of operational workers for immediate or near-term decision making (Inmon, Imhoff, and Battas, 1995). The data are volatile because they are updated continuously as old values are replaced, in contrast to the data warehouse, where none of the data are volatile but are time stamped and stored indefinitely.

The ODS assists integration in the operational environment and contains homogeneous, current detailed data. Metadata are helpful in this environment also. The data typically have a short time horizon and require a high-performance relational database management system (RDBMS). The ODS frequently becomes the system of record in environments with multiple legacy source applications that may be unintegrated. The system of record is the source of process control and the physical location for the deployment of business and clinical rules. Clinical rules may also be applied at the source, or original, applications. In health care, however, rules are frequently applied in cross-application analyses: for example, is it safe to administer a particular drug (pharmacy function) when a particular lab value is abnormal (laboratory function)?

Business rules are the assets of the health care enterprise. These are the rules that tend to differentiate the enterprise from the competition. In many cases they are a reflection of the standard of care. Differentiation rests in the organization's ability to execute them. In many other cases, however, rules are derived by local enterprises. They are frequently implemented through stored procedures on the transaction database server and may be portable through middleware standards. Frequently, they are applied best in the system of record, that is, across all OLTP applications in the enterprise.

The ODS may also be the source of process control, by automating and deploying rules that support point of care decision making for clinicians. This activity requires a high-performance response and uses a normalized relational data model.

An operational environment with multiple legacy applications using an ODS frequently requires conversion middleware, frequently referred to as an *interface engine*. In this case, middleware integrates the operational environment and functions between front-end applications and back-end domain servers of differing operating systems and technology platforms. Frequently, middleware offers a single point of control and serves a messaging function. Functionally, middleware may be viewed as client server *glue*, supporting integration and optimal performance in these environments.

Data Marts

The data mart is the "corner information store of the online enterprise within the integrated structure of the data warehouse (enterprise data store)" (Demarest, 1994). Data marts can serve as models for clinical workstations, facilitating clinical knowledge worker access to data warehouse information for on-line analytical processing—with simultaneous access to the ODS and OLTP systems—enabling an expeditious response to patient demands. (The information processing architecture, including the data warehouse, operational data store, and data marts, is presented in Figure 4.4.)

Data marts can accomplish OLAP with specific multidimensional analysis tools on a well-planned multidimensional data model. This is a high-performance on-line environment, employing relatively small amounts of data, which are periodically refreshed; enhanced with specific, predetermined analysis programs; and enabled for efficient access to ODS or data warehouse information employing a user-friendly metadata directory.

The data mart serves as an information tool with which clinical knowledge workers accomplish transactional duties such as order entry and clinical data entry. Data marts are ideal for the implementation of business or clinical rules through alerts, guidelines, reminders, parameters, calculations, and inferences executed out of the system of record. In addition, the data mart can offer OLAP for historical data, using preformatted analyses on pertinent clinical data that support analysis of historical trends and derivation of new business rules.

Management of the information processing architecture must address conception of the enterprise data model; data standardization and integration; performance of the technology platform in relation to processes, interfaces, and storage; development of the requirements definition process; decisions about data granularity and summarization; cost-benefit analysis; scalability for growth; decisions about business and clinical rules and the best way to deploy them; methods of reengineering workflow in the operational environment; and query and report coordination.

In the future the data mart, or clinical workstation, must support the following functions: computerized patient records (CPR), workflow automation, practice guidelines and care pathways, interaction checking processes, hypertext references, on-line resources (Internet, Medline, text formats), diagnostic processes, therapeutic processes, and drug dosing and prescription generation.

In summary, the information processing architecture development process requires the following steps:

1. Take inventory of information demands (external, internal).
2. Enlist clinical knowledge worker collaboration and input.
3. Standardize a structured vocabulary with precise definitions.
4. Conceive the information processing architecture and data model.
5. Derive and deploy business and clinical rules.
6. Design the data mart (clinical workstation) to support OLTP and OLAP for each particular knowledge worker.

In addition, Web-based architectures are highly desirable and facilitate distributed processing. The goals are to promote maximum user flexibility and optimization of network traffic. Processing capability may be distributed to the client for graphical presentation or manipulation, with the Web-based server housing the database system, search engine, and business logic.

Clinical Systems

Current nonautomated clinical systems are exemplified by the completion and movement of paperwork in a defined action sequence of reject, modify, or accept. Much redundancy is found in the creation of clinical documents, making the process tremendously inefficient and expensive. The environment is characterized by lack of pertinent information, lost and incomplete documents, lack of standardization of data elements, and tedious retrieval.

The goal of modern clinical systems is to eliminate clerical duties for the professional staff and all staff involved in the delivery of patient care. These duties are defined as those non-value-added tasks that simply sort, re-create, or store existing information.

There are several arguments supporting clinical automation. First and foremost, productivity suffers in the clinical setting and is probably most inefficient in the physician's office. Primary care physicians have estimated that 30 to 50 percent of their time is involved in clerical-type duties that are error prone and redundant (specialists estimate 15 to 50 percent) (personal survey). Another argument is that automation would reduce the tremendous variation in clinical processes and practice guidelines and supply alerting or reminding capabilities that are currently lacking for pending and important findings. Process improvements will require communication with many workers in the clinical setting and will be optimal only when these workers and the patient are included. Moreover, manual documentation probably results in less patient education and satisfaction during the specific encounter than is desirable. Finally, the necessity of profiling providers and linking performance to compensation is creating an impetus for clinical automation.

Generally, vendors involved in clinical systems employ two approaches. One is to "not disturb" the physician's work process. The other is to introduce innovative clinical work processes that include physicians' processes. Physicians, especially, should be looking toward the latter approach, because their participation and access to patients in managed care markets will probably be based on documented performance on clinical criteria that in all likelihood can be managed better by redesigned systems.

What are physicians looking for in office systems? They have identified as most important managed care contract tracking, access to information from multiple remote locations, decision support for potential interactions, reminders, outcomes measurements, reduction of manual repetitive tasks, reduction of malpractice liability, and presentation of focused flow sheets for active problems and health maintenance.

Physician product offerings consist of three distinct types of systems: practice management systems, clinical document systems, and workflow and decision support systems.

Practice management systems include such functions as registration, scheduling and reminders, billing, accounts receivable and ledger maintenance, electronic transmission, and financial reporting. These systems have traditionally been built around the metaphor of the financial batch. Generally, practices must maintain separate paper charts, although many established vendors are creating an accompanying clinical document system.

Clinical document systems focus on transcribing, word processing, and scanning. They frequently include images, document management tools, and reference interfaces to laboratory and other sources. Frequently, some have value-added features such as problem lists, medication lists, and drug interactions. Workflow features are limited and generally apply to only nonphysician staff. These packages may or may not have an associated practice management system. Outcomes analysis is generally limited to diagnoses

(ICD-9), billing codes (CPT), and free-text searches. These systems rely on a document metaphor for the electronic capture and retrieval of medical records. Frequently parallel paper charts are required.

Workflow and decision support systems are the most recent vendor offerings in the marketplace, and these products are still very much in development by start-up companies. They focus on clinical data capture as a by-product of the service and tend to be process based, using a structured medical vocabulary. The actions of physicians and all other clinical workers are automated. Guidelines are built into the process for interactive use. Data entry is intuitive and driven by *intelligent* templates, frequently using a knowledge base of clinical heuristics (rules) with executable knowledge, calculations, and inferences. This approach promotes linking outcomes to process and cost elements in some detail. Workflow and decision support systems often encompass other features of clinical documentation systems. They are not usually associated with practice management systems. Workflow and decision support systems use a workflow metaphor and do not require parallel paper charts.

These product offerings can be viewed as a spectrum, ranging from legacy systems (practice management systems) to status quo systems (clinical document systems), to innovative systems possibly offering competitive advantage (workflow and decision support systems) at the price of reengineering. Practice management systems may be characterized as low risk with limited clinical benefit. The products are mature, and no reengineering is required. Clinical document systems carry medium risk and benefits—with reasonable and mature products—and require relatively little reengineering. Workflow and decision support systems entail high risk and appreciably high potential benefits. They are currently represented by immature products and require major redesign of most clinical processes.

Why should physicians innovate and take risk? It is possible that productivity improvements will justify these risks, stabilizing clinical processes by reducing variation through implementation of clinical rules. Also outcomes and analysis reporting and resource management may be facilitated. If providers spend less time on non-value-added clerical activities, they will have more time to devote to health care delivery, possibly leading to improved satisfaction scores and retained market share.

The originator of the problem-oriented medical record, L. Weed, M.D., has stated that "no longer should providers practice medicine based only on what's in their head" (personal communication). Instead, the provider should use up-to-date information to the fullest, at the point of care, and in an interactive fashion. It is a given that in the future office automation products will integrate practice management (financial) and clinical systems. In all likelihood physicians will have nearly paperless offices, characterized by electronic health records, electronic data interchange (EDI), and e-mail. Diagnostic decision support and therapeutic decision support tools are very desirable, as are on-line medical textbooks, Medline, and continuing medical education. Outcomes tracking is necessary for payer contracting. Telemedicine as well may have great application if legal, reimbursement, and liability issues can be addressed.

In the future, technology such as handheld and wireless communication devices, voice recognition, handwriting recognition, patient information systems, and the Internet are expected to have significant impact in the clinical workplace.

Clinical workstations supporting clinical knowledge workers will be implemented incrementally. They must be intuitive, flexible, and high performance, guiding providers to structured medical vocabularies and practice guidelines. The goal is elimination of inappropriate variation in medical practice. The technical specifications of clinical workstations require an open systems (standards-based, nonproprietary) architecture. In addition, clinical users usually request the ability to enhance the features of applications locally with development kits or tool sets and the ability to construct ad hoc queries. Presumably they will also require high system reliability with no scheduled downtime. This necessitates disk mirroring and significant storage capabilities provided by employing a redundant array of inexpensive disks (RAID). Scalability of systems is extremely important, so systems can grow to handle the anticipated clinical load of thousands of patients in a highly granular data environment, tracking their information over several years.

Severity Systems

Severity systems measure an individual's inherent risk of a particular outcome and adjust for patient characteristics beyond the provider's control. In essence, they credit the best and brightest providers for taking care of the sickest and neediest patients, directly militating against cherry picking, that is, treating the healthiest patients in a prepaid plan. They document adverse selection for a provider or group and act as a control for the burden of illness at presentation. They are also useful for summarizing clinical progress in a complicated patient as the process of care continues. They apply to risks of adverse outcomes and expected resource use and are felt by many to be the cornerstone of outcomes management and clinical practice improvement (see, for example, Horn & Hopkins, 1994). Severity systems are known also as severity of illness systems, severity adjustment systems, morbidity-based case-mixed adjustment systems, and severity indexing systems. Severity systems are quite helpful for obtaining the risk-adjusted expected outcome and are critical for accurate provider profiling and performance-based compensation.

The importance of severity systems is exemplified by the Harvard Community Health Plan's use of a well-known ambulatory severity system, described in "When Good Apples Look Bad" (Salem-Schatz, Moore, Rucker, & Pearson, 1994). The authors note that failure to adjust for case mix in provider profiling may lead to overestimation of variation, misidentification of outliers ("good" bad apples and "bad" good apples), inequitable decisions and actions in relation to a provider's practice, and misdirection of scarce resources in an attempt to resolve nonproblems.

Several vendors' offerings are available for severity systems, with published studies documenting "goodness" of the model. Some of these systems focus on intensive care, acute care (hospital), or ambulatory care. Some are population based, episode based, or disease specific.

Development of a severity system is not an easy undertaking. Pertinent risk factors with discrete definitions must be determined. Appropriate data sources, including administrative or clinical data elements, must be identified. Next, decisions must be made on the timing of data element collection and the methodology, along with the rules for data quality control. Most severity systems have constructed stratified risk models, often with rigorous statistical regression techniques based on thousands of patient histories. For widespread acceptance a severity model must be validated in different populations with appropriate attention to comparative performance and statistical certainty (reflected in confidence intervals).

In summary, the characteristics of an ideal severity system are that it is disease specific, independent of treatments, comprehensive, clinically credible, able to measure outcomes along the care continuum (ambulatory, acute, and intensive care), and statistically valid. The ability to score various psychosocial elements is also felt to be important, especially in ambulatory settings (Horn & Hopkins, 1994). A more detailed discussion of adjusting for severity is presented in Chapter Eight.

Patient-Provider Systems

Patient information systems in the form of informative textbooks have been available for some time. The Internet has now brought the potential of greatly facilitated patient-provider communication, foreseeing a much closer relationship than previously known.

In some of these systems, patients are virtually interconnected directly to providers through the Internet or direct dial-up. In this way, guidelines can be extended to the home, and compliance can be effectively measured. These systems are reasonably economical and have been found to be a great facilitator of patient satisfaction. There is some evidence that they might even reduce malpractice liability.

By employing a system such as this when much of the value and control in health care delivery has accumulated in the employer-plan relationship, it is quite possible to return the value to the patient-provider relationship. For this reason such communication between providers and patients should be very attractive to PCCOs.

Applications Supporting Coordinated Care

Interactive voice response systems for patient self-education have great potential in demand management programs. Telephone triage systems employing various trained health care providers can also be an integral part of demand management systems, which are increasingly taking a proactive approach. Disease management systems clearly recommend preventive contact with patients at high risk of progression and manifestation of established diseases such as diabetes and asthma. Case management systems have typically been retrospective in their approach, to limit catastrophic costs associated with costly diagnoses (such as AIDS), but they also have proven useful in coordinating care for the desperately ill. Home health and home infusion systems can be quite supportive of coordinated care organizations, and communication between home providers, primary physicians, and specialists could be critical in optimizing the home care setting. Protocol systems have great potential. Through them physicians may leverage their skills and talents and reach (via midlevel providers) pharmaceutical care providers, respiratory therapists, physical therapists, and occupational therapists.

Enterprise Communications

E-mail is a standard offering in most health care delivery systems, although it is still poorly used by many physicians. Groupware, with its discussion database, workflow automation, and application development tools, can clearly go beyond standard e-mail in facilitating provider collaboration. For example, many of the time and distance limitations on meetings can be overcome with groupware. Such on-line meetings may be used by pools of providers to discuss quality improvement and resource management for the patients they manage. Considering the need for collaboration among so many providers in coordinated care, groupware becomes an attractive option.

The Internet—with e-mail, scheduling, conferencing, groupware features, and even clinical systems—may have tremendous implications for collaboration within PCCOs. Several advanced clinical systems at well-known academic medical centers are presently executed over the Internet. Increasingly, clinical systems vendors are looking at the Internet as a distribution channel for their particular product. The economics of distributing a clinical application over the Internet are very favorable when compared with provider-by-provider installation and support.

Intranets are closed, secure networks that use Internet (and World Wide Web) development and access tools. They have a promising future, especially where there is concern about Internet security, performance, or the political correctness of making the uncensored Internet available to all in the corporate environment. Videoconferencing and telemedicine are going to play important roles in distributed systems, especially those involving rural physicians.

Managed Care Information Systems

Managed care contracting has put significant demands on practice management systems from a physician's perspective. First and foremost, comparing fee-for-service revenue with capitated contracts is of interest in a transitioning marketplace. Maintaining eligibility information and the master member index is critical but not easily accomplished without accurate and timely transmissions from payers. The ability to track patient encounters by CPT, payer, and cost is critical for decision making concerning the profitability of a given plan for the provider. Electronic claims submission is mandatory. The ability to track plan benefits across multiple plans coordinated with electronic posting of explanation of benefits is important to determine if appropriate payments are being received in return for services. Payers also put significant importance on HEDIS compliance. It is considerably more efficient for a physician's office to maintain electronic records of such compliance than for the payer to do so, especially for some of the preventive maintenance schedules. Such systems invariably lead to improved alerts and reminders for compliance with suggested regimens.

Employers want managed care information systems that can report on provider performance and facilitate focused management reporting that conveys information for decision support. Employers like to see evidence that various patient management options are considered in the delivery of health care. It is also desirable to link utilization review of prospective decisions with adjudication, quality management, and case management. Employers are increasingly concerned about parameters that reflect expenditures such as hospital days, emergency room visits, and pharmaceutical expenses.

Traditional needs managed care information systems have centered on eligibility, benefit design, member co-pays and deductibles, provider credentialing, type of service, and diagnosis. Problems experienced in these systems have been payment of duplicate claims, payment for services not covered, overpayments, and payment for ineligible members. Strategic issues in managed care information systems at the present time involve plan accountability, profitability assessment, robust plan benefit design, and compliance with budget forecasting. Many managed care plans have abundant data, but accurate information is extremely rare. Plans of the future will require information that is available, usable, and valid and that can be obtained efficiently at minimal expense.

Internal efficiency measures for PCCOs are mandatory for future competitiveness and include performance profiling of providers, groups, institutions, and plans; reliable cost estimates; simulation and forecasting modeling scenarios; cost savings and risk pool management; and contract administration (Ruffin, 1995).

Managed care information systems must also support external reporting, detailing enrollee demographics, claims paid and claims incurred, and comparisons to norms and standards and offering catastrophic case monitoring, provider reports, benefits modeling, variance reports, and HEDIS reporting. Progressive managed care information systems vendors are focusing development on comorbidity and case-mix indexing, provider profiling with comparisons to benchmarks, prior authorization processes for referrals and institutions, concurrent review processes, claims processing that includes adjudication, repricing for discounted fee schedules, funds management for bonus pools, capitation rate calculation, number of lives enrolled calculation, practice capacity calculation, tracking of date of enrollment and disenrollment, and contract compliance audits.

Future systems will focus on severity-adjusted quality assessment and management, with improved granularity of clinical events enabling outcomes analysis that links outcomes to process and cost. Likewise, resource management using activity-based costing and management techniques will be employed, allowing non-value-added activities to be eliminated and cost variances to be understood and monitored. Provider incentive compensation will be tied to performance on quality and resource management. In the future, point-of-care decision making through guidelines and reminders (as opposed to the retrospective oversight methodologies) will be the norm.

PCCOs can focus their attention on four areas when considering requirements for systems development or acquisition: member services, provider services, claim processing and funds management, and quality and resource management.

Member Services

Member services will be an area of critical functionality for coordinated care organizations as they attempt to develop brand name recognition among their patients. Member services may evolve away from the insurance plan sponsor and be delivered through the coordinated care organization. The master member index confirming eligibility and enrollment is a critical component of such systems. Member registration and scheduling of various care-delivery encounters, ensuring appropriate access to care, are keys to success. Preventive maintenance reminders to patients and their providers and demand management programs encompassing self-care, counseling, and advice triage will all support care coordination. Both member complaints resolution and patient satisfaction assessment should be integrated with member services. Moreover, it is important to match the geographical distribution of members with available providers and to offer members referral services.

Provider Services

Member referral and assignment coordinated with geographical assessment of provider capacity are important aspects of a provider services system. Other important functions are maintaining a record of the credentialing, qualifications, capabilities, and capacity of individual providers; tracking provider contracts and recredentialing requirements; appraising provider distribution by specialty; and marketing provider capacity and distribution to payers and purchasers. Recruiting needed and qualified providers is a function of provider services. Information on the health status of the community of patients served, as a measure of provider performance, will also eventually be shared with payers and employers for marketing purposes.

Claims Processing and Funds Management

Electronic data interchange between providers and a claims processing hub is effective and efficient. Adjudication, or validation of previous utilization decisions, is critical. Coordination of benefits with other payers, such as Medicare or Worker's Compensation, is consequently a characteristic of an efficient and timely claims payment or issuance system. It is vital for provider satisfaction and ongoing support.

Funds management in prepaid risk-sharing agreements is essential and includes capitation rate calculation and fee-for-service (equivalence) estimation. Tracking for per diems, stop loss reinsurance, withhold pools, and savings pools is sometimes elaborate and requires significant flexibility for multiple plans. Other key areas to track are incurred but not reported encounters, co-pays and deductibles, grace period funds, and network funds. Contract administration is key to negotiating and maintaining contracts for prepaid care, as are cost forecasting, budgeting, and simulation.

Quality and Resource Management

Encounter tracking and forecasting, along with authorization and referral management (prior, concurrent, and retrospective), are key elements of a quality improvement and resource management system. Provider profiling, including data on patient satisfaction, access to care, functional status, outcomes, and utilization, is mandatory in this prepaid environment. Decision support systems for appropriateness soon will be deployed at the point of care, to be used before decisions are made.

Proactive outcomes management relies on severity adjustment systems and standardization of various coding schemes for diagnosis, procedures, and process (ICD-9, CPT, SNOMED). Other clinical systems for order entry, results reporting, electronic global health records, practice guidelines, and decision support at the point of care are essential for deploying business and clinical rules.

Decision support systems at the point of care, invoking alerts, reminders, calculations, and inferences, are within the realm of quality management systems. Disease state management and case management systems, propagating guidelines as well as functional status indices assessment (SF 36), are also indispensable components of an outcomes management system.

Enterprise Performance

Organizational performance can best be monitored through attention to certain key measures known as the dashboard (Luttman, Siren, & Laffel, 1994) or balanced scorecard (Kaplan & Norton, 1996a). The dashboard of organizational performance may be assessed from three perspectives: customer, financial, and operational. An appropriate customer dashboard includes market share, profitability, payer satisfaction, provider satisfaction, hospital days per thousand members per year, member plan satisfaction, and member community health status. Dashboards for the financial perspective include indicators of adequate capital, debt service coverage ratios, cash flow, liquidity, plan profitability (net, gross profit margin), forecasting reliability, return on investment, severity-adjusted cost per member, medical expense and administrative load ratios, and medical cost determination (primary care physician, specialist, hospital, pharmacy) (Coyne, 1993). The dashboard for the operational perspective relates to outcomes, adverse events, guideline variance, utilization per thousand members per year, productivity per full-time equivalent, staff satisfaction survey, percentage of board-certified physicians, and access to care measures.

Functional Interdependence

There are many examples of the interdependence among the various managed care functions. For example, quality resource management preauthorization data are used by claims processing during adjudication. Member services benefit design data are used by quality and resource management in preauthorization determinations. Member service satisfaction and access to care data are used by quality resource management for provider profiling. Member services care coordination services are also used by quality resource management preauthorization, and likewise, care coordination services rely on quality resource management appropriateness and triage guidelines. Quality and resource management preauthorization relies on provider services accreditation and capabilities assessment. Funds management relies on provider services contracting information for appropriate disbursement. Provider services recruiting relies on member services distribution information. Outcomes management relies on member services care coordination for optimizing efficient health care delivery.

Systems Analysis, Design, and Implementation

It is recommended that a structured methodology such as the SDLC be employed in any systems acquisition. The SDLC approach is characterized by documented deliverables at each of the seven phases in the process. Management initially sets the goals and budget, and users define the system during joint application development sessions and with the use of specified modeling tools. The phases in the SDLC consist of planning, when management determines feasibility and strategic value; analysis, to identify end-user requirements, using modeling tools such as entity relationship and data flow diagrams; general design, analyzing input, output, processes, database, technology, and security and controls requirements; systems evaluation and selection, involving a comparative cost-benefit evaluation; detailed design, culminating in the explicit description of the requirements noted under general design along with creation of an RFP; systems implementation, relying heavily on project management in a postimplementation project; and systems maintenance, in which maintenance work order, quality improvement, and formal change management systems are addressed.

Cost-Benefit Analysis and Vendor Selection

A formalized cost-benefit analysis is beneficial in defining expected benefits and costs (Gilbreath, Nelson, Schilp, & Burch, 1996). Although this exercise may not be entirely predictive, it increases organizational members' understanding of the expected benefits and costs. Vendors should have significant input into this process.

Benefits may be tangible or intangible. Tangible benefits generally involve productivity, such as a reduction in the need for full-time equivalents (FTEs) or increased productivity per FTE, and are generally easy to measure. Intangible benefits entail differentiation, such as increased market share, and manageability of operations, such as the ability to reduce cycle time or improve resource scheduling. These should not be ignored and can have extremely high financial benefits.

Costs generally encompass three areas: hardware, software, and personnel (including retraining or hiring personnel with a new skill set).

Capital budgeting calculates the expected financial return adjusted to the present value through three well-defined techniques:

- Net present value: this calculation generally has the advantage of being accurate but is presented in a way (dollar value) that may not be intuitively pleasing.

- Internal rate of return: this calculation gives a pleasing and intuitive rate of return but may suffer from inaccuracies, especially if the flow of cash is inconsistent.

- Marginal return on invested capital: this calculation has the advantage of being accurate and producing a rate of return but is quite complicated to calculate.

Request for Proposal

An RFP to information systems vendors is ideally contractually binding and outlines specific requirements for the job at hand. Using an RFP is generally recommended unless the market is well established and an off-the-shelf purchase can be made for a well-defined and standard process. The vendor that promises to "provide what you need in the future" sometimes has significant hidden costs and a less than optimum interpretation of what is needed.

The RFP does not need to be unduly complicated or long. It serves the purpose of aligning the expectations of both vendor and organizational members. The SDLC methodology is often a good starting point for creating an RFP. This process should be user driven, so that functional requests are delineated, technical requirements are understood, and an implementation plan for scheduling and staffing is outlined. Other information obtained in an RFP includes vendor customer referrals, the financial position of the vendor, and price and payment options.

When evaluating vendors, organizations should assess such important aspects as vendor platform acceptability, functionality match, track record of installation and support, market share, position on the product life cycle, personnel profile, economic stability, and implementation schedule and price options. An analysis of the staff the vendor employs in the areas of marketing, development, support, and management can reveal how much emphasis is placed on those respective functions.

Conclusion

PCCOs should take an inventory of information demands in the critical areas of quality, resource, and outcomes management and standardize the data elements and definitions as the enterprise data model. The focus must be on internal and external reporting requirements, as ultimately the data model must expedite clinical practice improvement initiatives.

In designing systems the SDLC methodology has the advantages of documented deliverables and a well-proven methodology for outlining requirements put forth in an RFP, which is indispensable for vendor evaluation and selection. Employing these techniques ensures a user-driven process that has the best chance of implementing the complex requirements of PCCOs.

Chapter Six

Information-Driven Medical Management

Roy E. Gilbreath
Judy Lawing

Medical management driven by clinical and
financial performance information has many
advantages. It allows physicians and other
providers to view their patients objectively in the
context of population health and to assess their
own performance through its positive effects on the
health of the population of patients they serve.
This chapter reviews strategic concepts in
attaining this vision: assessment of clinical value
opportunities, continuous quality improvement,
and coordination of care. It also discusses tactical
approaches to enhance the health of patients
served: physician support alliances,
interdisciplinary clinical work teams, project
management, clinical measurement and
quantitative analysis, benchmarking, and
communication and innovation.

A medical management program should be centered on a true
concern for quality as well as cost. Physicians and other providers
of care, who affect the majority of the discretionary resources

consumed, will simply not have it any other way. Medical professionals will not accept cost reduction programs unless they are intricately and tightly linked to a positive impact on quality and patient outcomes.

One way to link quality and cost is through assessment of clinical value opportunities. In health care delivery, value is often defined using the value equation shown in Figure 1.1.

As the equation shows, quality and access are directly proportional and are positively correlated to value, while cost is indirectly proportional or negatively correlated with value. Quality includes both medical content and service. It is easy to see why medical professionals relate to the value equation. Any intervention delivered in the course of patient care has a certain quality as well as cost implications. Medical professionals intrinsically grasp the potential trade-offs between quality and cost and wish to ensure the highest quality in every case.

Physicians especially relate well to the notion of clinical value improvement. This notion offers the possibility of objective recognition of the intangibles in medical practice such as bedside manner.

Definitions

Some clarifications are needed at this point to describe certain terms used throughout this discussion. *Medical management* is the set of interventions that are applied to (1) improve the health of the target population and (2) mitigate the financial risk for health care costs that are inherent in that population. *Performance improvement* diligently examines current practices and, with process interventions, measures progress toward an objective level of achievement.

Care management is the application of appropriate preventative and health maintenance interventions that ultimately improve the target population's health. *Disease management* is a facet of care management that focuses on certain high-risk disease states with programmatic interventions designed to improve access and quality and reduce unnecessary costs. *Demand management,* another facet, implements interventions in the general population, as well as certain disease states, that, in fact, improve patient access to care intentionally, at an earlier time in the disease process, with the goal of reducing the demand that occurs in patients without the intervention. *Care coordination* involves examining all the relevant aspects that have an impact on patient choice (psychological, social, economic, medical, etc.) and, considering medical necessity, optimizes the placement of the patient to the right provider, setting, and ultimately intensity of level of care.

Clinical effectiveness measures the ability to deliver what was intended by certain known clinical processes and interventions. It measures the effects and efficiency of a delivery process or intervention in a target population. *Physician and provider profiling* measures individual performance and variation from a benchmark of a key clinical parameter. In provider-sponsored organizations, these individual profiles are known only to the subject and not released for public or peer knowledge.

The Culture of Continuous Quality Improvement

Successful medical management programs, in applying a set of interventions designed to improve the health of the target population and reduce that population's risk for health care costs, encompass the basic principles of continuous quality improvement (CQI) (Longo, 1988). CQI is a philosophy of management that strives to improve performance through the exclusion of poor quality during production or delivery of the product or service, rather than relying on an ability to correct problems afterward. CQI establishes process specifications, measures performance, and determines inappropriate variation. One of the key concepts is the elimination of *quality waste,* quality failures that result in higher costs. Process redesign seeks to design in quality, eliminating unnecessary variation. As one cycle of improvement ends, another ensues, thereby ensuring a continuous effort to enhance performance. Central to this approach is worker empowerment, which drives out fear of reprisal and under which "killing the messenger" of unfavorable performance data is not allowed.

CQI also delineates and clarifies the customer relationship, making that relationship paramount for aligning efforts within the organization. Patient-derived scales or surveys addressing satisfaction, functional status, and health-related quality of life become important outcomes of care in addition to standard medical outcomes such as mortality, complications, and success rates. Industrial methods such as statistical process control employing standard control chart methodology to assess common cause (random) variation and special cause (system) variation are used. Benchmarking, internally or externally, to best practices is a key component of this tactical approach to provider standardization, process improvement, and change in practices.

The focus of CQI should be the health of the target population served rather than individual performance. *Bad apple*-seeking behavior has proven inhibitory to true collaboration and process innovation. In an environment of fear, performance measurement is driven underground because individuals' status in the organization is not dependent on creativity, innovation, and performance but on politicization, clique membership, and momentum in pointing the finger first.

A key aspect of the CQI philosophy is the relationship between quality and cost, viewed through the concept of quality waste. Quality failures are frequently a result of poorly designed systems or processes of production or delivery, and typically have major cost implications because of the rework required.

A focus on population health takes attention off individual case review and places it on understanding trends, summary information, and statistical significance. Appropriate understanding of the health status of the population in terms of severity of illness and expected outcome and cost is critical from the provider perspective. Suitable utilization of severity systems guards against penalizing the best and brightest physicians and providers for taking care of the sickest and neediest patients.

Organizational Infrastructure

Health care delivery organizations may approach medical management from many different organizational structure perspectives. Most experts have recommended a decentralized structure, simply because it emphasizes the empowerment of the frontline providers and workers in direct contact with patients. Typical system-level functions related to medical management are (1) performance and quality improvement; (2) Joint Commission on Accreditation of Healthcare Organizations (JCAHO) and National Committee for Quality Assurance (NCQA) regulatory adherence; (3) clinical and financial decision support; (4) clinical measurement and quantitative analysis; (5) coordinated care (disease, case, outcome, and utilization management and social services); (6) orientation of service lines around functional patient groupings; (7) information technology and systems; and (8) a balanced scorecard system. Organizations must meet the infrastructural requirements of these supporting structures in order to adequately facilitate an organizational improvement philosophy.

The performance and quality improvement function typically provides the priorities, process, standards, and facilitators for efforts in this endeavor. Policies and procedures are standardized for the purpose of enabling comparisons of projects' benefits and costs. Improvement project resources are finite, and priorities must be set based on mission, vision, core competencies, and relative opportunities for improvement. Indeed, an opportunity assessment of existing service lines (see addendum) often reveals surprises in terms of where efforts and resources should be focused to have the largest gain.

Accreditation bodies (JCAHO and NCQA) require certain performance reporting simply for health care providers to be in the game. Initiatives such as the Health Care Financing Administration

(HCFA) CQI projects (CQIP) or Health Plan Employer Data and Information Set (HEDIS) participation must be addressed seriously and consistently because of their public disclosure and regulatory requirements. Most organizations designate one or several full-time equivalents (FTEs) to specifically address these requirements.

Clinical and financial decision support systems may reside in several areas, including information services, financial accounting, and clinical areas such as performance improvement and clinical measurement and quantitative analysis. The key is clinical-financial data integration in order to best address the value equation and identify quality and cost opportunities for improvement.

Clinical measurement and quantitative analysis are common functions within provider systems today. They enable the appropriate manipulation, analysis, and presentation of data for the purposes of medical management. Frequently, design of projects is undertaken by these functions also. Use of very large databases for medical management is commonplace, as is supplementation with data abstracted from the medical record. Several issues arise with abstracted data that require statistical purview, including interrater reliability, data element validity and consistency, data collection expense, and terminology standardization.

Clinical measurement programs typically employ senior statisticians and require considerable expertise in graphical presentation of information, unlike decision support departments, which typically provide data in tables without postulating statistical significance.

A new organizational approach is the coordinated care department, which is made up of merged entities from utilization management, social services, and outcomes coordinators (clinical nurse specialists). This department functions on the concept of *care management,* which takes an encompassing view of health care system resources. This approach decreases fragmentation of services and facilitates proactive planning for care management and patient transition from one intensity level of care to another. These limited health care system resources are ordinarily deployed on the target population of patients, and frequently the organization has some form of financial risk involved. Coordinated care departments blend appropriateness of care and medical necessity with an emphasis on outcomes management, prevention of adverse events, and improvement of the functional status and satisfaction of patients and customer physicians. Coordinated care is the functional implementation of the adage, "provide the patient with the right care at the right time and place, and to the right degree."

The coordinated care concept is a strategy that organizes and manages patient care. Traditionally, fragmentation of care resulted from specialization of services. Coordinated care incorporates case management principles to coordinate all components of care and to facilitate the ongoing evaluation of patient progress. Positive results include decreased fragmentation of care, decreased duplication of services, increased interdisciplinary collaboration, and increased coordination of care and resources.

This concept facilitates the operationalization of continuous quality improvement in the clinical setting. Proactive management of care-related processes positively affects both financial and clinical outcomes. Along with effective communication, it can contribute toward appropriate length of stay and resource utilization, patient, patient family, and staff satisfaction, and multidisciplinary collaboration. It evaluates in real time the components of the quality circle: appropriate practice, efficient process, and effective outcome.

Initial organization of a coordinated care department should involve all areas whose departments will be affected by the integration. Essential processes are defined, and accountability is assigned to the newly defined roles. Departments usually involved in this reorganization are utilization management, case management, outcomes management, and social work services. A clear mission and vision for the new department is critical to support changes that will affect not just the individual associates whose roles have been redefined but the entire organization.

Clinical pathways are an effective tool to support the coordinated care structure. Pathways specific to particular populations can be used for case types that have predictable patterns of care. Used as a multidisciplinary plan of care, pathways standardize the outcomes approach to care and also standardize documentation of that care. The pathway also defines who is accountable for components of care and on what part of the expected timeline those interventions or outcomes should occur. Generic pathways are useful for those patients who are less predictable or who are not high-volume case types. Participation by physicians from the very beginning of a pathway initiative is critical to its success.

Pathways provide a tool for concurrent monitoring of care and facilitate the redirection of clinical activities in response to patient progress or lack of progress. Selective indicators from the pathways can be used to track and trend process or utilization concerns. Outcomes indicators can be incorporated to evaluate cause-and-effect relationships between interventions or processes and optimal outcomes.

Programs in disease management for certain diagnosed populations and in wellness and demand management for the general target populace are integral components of coordinated care. Disease management is a set of standard guidelines and interventions used with a known population of patients with a certain condition, whose outcomes can be significantly influenced by compliance with recommendations. It has been applied to conditions such as diabetes, asthma and chronic obstructive pulmonary disease, congestive heart failure, somatization and stress management, and acquired immunodeficiency syndrome.

Patients are educated on common disease manifestations and issues in management and are enrolled in a support program, ensuring their early access to care in an effort to halt progression or prevent complications of the condition. Pre- and postintervention cost-benefit analyses are important aspects of disease management programs.

Wellness and demand management is applied to the whole population of patients served in an effort to apply standard, well-accepted preventive care, and facilitate access to providers for advice, recommendations, and appropriate scheduling. It relies heavily on telephonic interplay and may have certain proactive provisions to help ensure wellness in the target population.

Service line orientation around functional patient groupings greatly promotes medical management and performance improvement efforts. Rigid professionalism, a departmental orientation, and turf issues often constrain the implementation of services that would fit customers and patients better. Service line approaches typically allow flexibility within a given domain, and surprising synergies can arise between units aligned in meeting service line goals and objectives.

Information technology, provided by information systems and services departments, obviously plays a major role in medical management initiatives. Communication to providers about standards, guidelines, and performance is critical, and in the future an Internet-based means of providing this communication is likely to be used. Maintenance of very large databases of clinical and financial information is key to successful information systems, and these databases require significant resources to maintain. Deployment of point-of-care reminders through order entry and results reporting systems is the ultimate manifestation of proactive medical management; standards and guidelines will be more readily available, and staff will not have to memorize them or do off-line research to decipher them. Fault-tolerant, high-performing hardware and technology, including network platforms, are absolutely critical. Disaster contingency planning, especially for systems affecting clinical information flow, is of paramount importance.

Balanced scorecard systems are described by Kaplan and Norton (1996a). The balanced scorecard is a performance management methodology designed to align an organization around its strategic mission, vision, and values. The tactical application of the organization's goals and objectives is reflected in the balanced scorecard measurement system, which shows the performance expectations of every management level as well as of the frontline workers. This requires that performance measures cascade throughout the hierarchy of workers and that individual performance criteria roll up to a summary that becomes the performance measure for the accountable manager. The balanced scorecard is enabled and effective only when fully automated, requiring significant information technology services and support. Multiple legacy information systems must be interfaced with the balanced scorecard system to obtain the full benefits and efficiencies. (See also the case discussion on balanced scorecards in Chapter Thirteen.)

Organizational Structure

The organizational structure to support medical management and performance improvement must offer governance, authority, and accountability over the effort (see Figure 6.1 for a generic example).

The board of trustees has ultimate responsibility for the financial viability and clinical quality of the health system. The board performance council, reporting to the board of trustees, can prioritize initiatives, review summary results, and determine strategic goals.

The system quality council, at least half of whose membership should be physicians, determines the tactical approaches toward the goals of performance improvement, prioritizing, setting objectives, and reviewing results on specific improvement projects. The administrative executive council and the medical staff executive committee receive relevant reports and requests from the system quality council. Medical management and performance improvement initiatives are created, deployed, and executed through the service line interactive planning boards, which facilitate unit-based initiatives, appoint team members, arrange synergies, and institute permanent process changes as appropriate. Likewise, service line units assemble self-directed work teams, tasked with domain-specific process improvements, and rely heavily on collaboration, creativity, and innovation. Physicians have key leadership roles at all

Figure 6.1. Generic Medical Management and Performance Improvement (MM/PI) Governance.

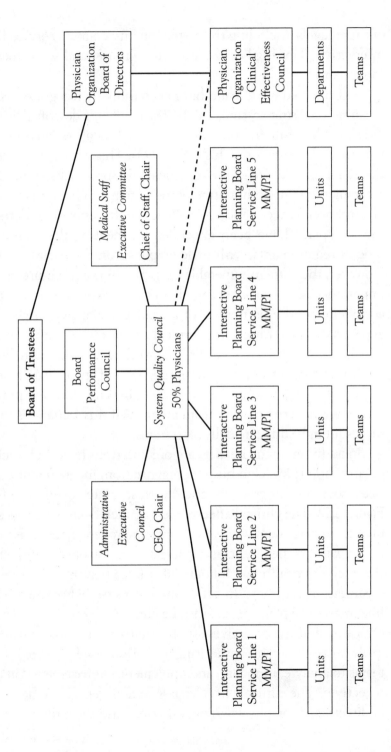

of these levels, including the system quality council, service line interactive planning boards, unit work groups, and self-directed work teams.

Self-directed work teams have been formally recognized as an organizational strategy since the 1940s, after being described by the Tavistock Institute in London as "sociotechnical systems design" (Maxwell, Zeigenfuss, & Chisholm, 1993). This strategy recognizes the equal importance of the technical and social subsystems and recommends joint optimization of the systems to obtain maximum organizational effectiveness and efficiency. Traditionally, efforts in the workplace have been expended on meeting the technical process requirements, with little emphasis on the social system. However, there are innumerable examples in the literature of the importance of the social ensemble in the workplace. Taking into consideration the particulars of a unique social system enables appropriate matching of technical requirements and social processes. Autonomous, self-directed work teams will often effectively implement this jointly optimized work if appropriate incentives, authority, boundaries, and accountability are instituted. Physicians are critical work team members if this scenario is to be successful in health care delivery systems.

In addition, many health care organizations have a physician organization (physician hospital organization, independent practice association, or group practice) with separate governance (see Figure 6.1). The clinical effectiveness council deals with issues of medical management and performance improvement as it pertains to the patients the physician organization is responsible for; often this includes dealing with financial risk for health maintenance organization contracts. In action analogous to that of the service line interactive planning boards, the clinical effectiveness council prioritizes and sets objectives for physician organization units (frequently departments), authorizing formation of self-directed work teams to analyze, innovate, and implement improvements on the objectives. The clinical effectiveness council reports to the board of directors of the physician organization, and these directors are linked to the system board of trustees. Frequent collaboration and cross-reporting to the system quality council occurs around shared initiatives.

The health system organizational structure reflects the execution of process changes required by medical management and performance improvement initiatives and validated by the governance authorities. Figure 6.2 illustrates a conventional organizational structure diagram, with the chief executive officer (CEO) reporting to the board of trustees. The CEO has five senior executives: the chief financial officer (CFO), chief strategy officer (CSO), chief operating officer (COO), chief medical officer (CMO), and chief information officer (CIO). Various functions are distributed among these five executive areas, optimizing strengths and synergies among them. This structure distributes the medical management and performance improvement infrastructure needs among all senior executives, placing a premium on collaboration, coordination, and communication among them to optimally support clinical and financial improvement projects.

In summary, it is organizational governance (authority and accountability) and organizational structure (execution) that enable an effectual medical management and performance improvement program.

Medical Management: A Tactical Approach

A world-class health system must establish the medical management and performance improvement strategic vision and objectives, instill the CQI culture and philosophy, and install organizational governance and structure.

There are six tactics in particular that organizations can employ to realize the benefits of a medical management and performance improvement program:

- Physician support alliances
- Interdisciplinary clinical work teams

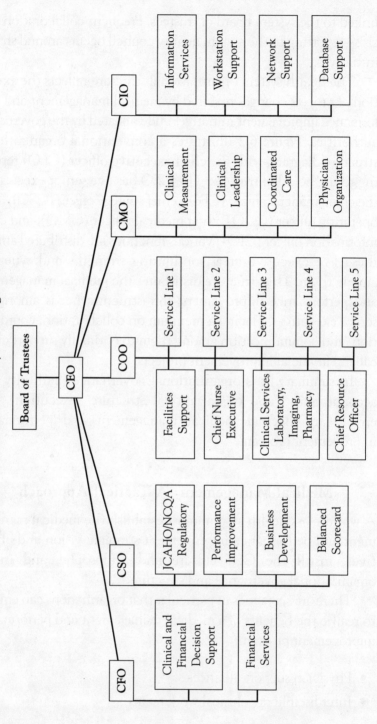

Figure 6.2. Generic Health System Organizational Structure.

- Project management
- Clinical measurement and quantitative analysis
- Benchmarking
- Communication and innovation

Physician Support Alliances

Clinical leadership is a prerequisite for medical management and performance improvement. An alliance must be created with the relevant physicians, whether the alliance is solidified or diffuse. The vast objective of identifying and establishing a relationship with each of the relevant individual physicians is daunting, so an approach that cultivates in-depth relationships with the designated or suspected physician opinion leaders is preferred. Remember, the informal influence of opinion leaders may be more significant than the formal leadership of the elected medical staff officers and medical directors.

The goal of clinical leadership is to manage clinical change, or more positively stated, to facilitate innovation in practice patterns toward organizational goals, which are ideally shared by and mutually beneficial to physicians, hospitals, and the delivery system. Clinical integration is the process by which physicians are allied, consulted, empowered, and held accountable for the system performance, as well as their own performance. Integration is not easy to attain and occurs as physicians come to believe that they are valued participants, have some influence, are achieving mutual benefits, are realizing enhanced outcomes for their patients, and possess a trusting relationship with health system leaders, executives, and the board.

Financial incentives outside of risk-sharing arrangements have many legal pitfalls and must be carefully designed to comply with the changing regulations in this area. Specifically, for Medicare and Medicaid patients, Stark Fraud and Abuse Regulations prohibit "payment for referrals" and any financial incentives for limiting services. *Gainsharing*—sharing of savings generated by utilization management with physicians—was once popular but now appears to have fallen into disfavor by the Office of Inspector General as an "inducement to limit services to beneficiaries" and may be prosecuted.

Nonfinancial incentives can be very effective and relate to status and recognition rewards, program enhancement funding, co-branding joint physician and facility services, and educational support forums. If effects by work teams, including physicians, result in significant system savings, a portion of these savings may be designated to a fund for program enhancement that has major input from the participating physicians. Program enhancement funding operates within certain boundaries and can typically be applied to clinical information management, educational programs, and branding of clinical programs.

An aspect of creating physician support alliances is to manage the diffusion of innovations in physician cultures. The body of medical science, and therefore the standard of care, is in a constant state of flux. Evidence-based clinical innovations occur at an astounding pace. Equally important are process-based innovations that may be created in local institutions and may even contribute to the organization's trade secrets. The facilitation of the diffusion of these innovations in the social system, particularly with physicians, is complex.

Diffusion in organizations, as defined by Rogers (1995), is the "process by which an innovation is communicated through certain channels over time among the members of a social system or organization." Diffusion is in essence individual behavior change in a social context. Innovations represent creative solutions for dealing with change and have varying degrees of uncertainty associated with them. Thus, embracing change and adopting an innovation is inherently risky and troublesome for the individual because of the education, effort, and reestablishment of social connections that may be required.

The most critical aspect of the diffusion process is its initial 10 to 20 percent, when the early adopters are embracing the particular innovation. The opinion leaders among the early adopters are the deciding factor in diffusion, because once they are on board, the diffusion is likely to be completed.

Opinion leaders may also be the formally chosen leaders, but they are frequently informally appointed by the members of the social system. Much of their leadership is exerted through the grapevine. They have the ability to lead change through early personal adoption. Once their support of innovations perceived to be successful in the past is recognized, they are frequently reselected to opinion leadership status in the face of ongoing innovations. They have a knack for diplomacy, avoid alienating a majority of colleagues and other staff, and are recognized as maintaining the system norms. They typically have an exquisite talent for reinvention of the innovation in a way that incorporates the peculiarities of the organization's unique social system. As a result of this reinvention, a given innovation may better fit the adopter organization's specific situation.

The various adopter roles in an organization are innovators (less than 5 percent), early adopters (approximately 15 percent), early majority (32 percent), late majority (32 percent), and laggards (16 percent).

The characteristics that vary across adopter roles involve economic status, risk tolerance, intergroup network, cosmopolite (external) network, group social status, creativity, and traditionality. Most opinion leaders are in the early adopter category and tend to have high intergroup connectedness and position, moderate traditionality, and demonstrably high economic status and are moderately risk tolerant, creative, and cosmopolite. Innovators themselves typically have lower economic and group status, high risk tolerance and creativity, low intergroup networking and traditionality, and higher external networking. The early majority tend to have high intergroup networking, low creativity, and moderate economic and group status, external networking, traditionality, and risk tolerance. The late majority have high traditionality and economic status, medium intergroup networking and group status, and low external exposure, risk tolerance, and creativity. Laggards are risk aversive and demonstrate little creativity, with little intergroup networking or external exposure. They usually are of high economic status, moderate group status, and are so prominently traditional, they can serve as the historians for the organization.

Several variables determine the rate of diffusion of a given innovation in an organization. Among them, one set concerns the innovation itself: its relative advantage over the status quo, its compatibility with the values of the organization, the complexity of adapting to it, its ability to be pilot tested, and the observability of superior results attributable explicitly to the innovation.

Another variable in the rate of adoption is the type of the innovation decision: is it collective or authoritative or is it optional? The characteristics of the communication channels are important, with personal interplay more influential than impersonal mass media. The social system norms are significant, with risk-taking, openness of participation, creativity, and empowerment favoring adoption and politicization, risk aversion, and hierarchical management working against it. Finally, the extent of change agent promotion efforts is crucial and frequently a variable that can be capitalized on by management.

Change agents facilitate the adoption of innovations usually by (1) establishing the existence of a performance gap (difference between worst and best performers) or other impending threat to the organization, (2) establishing information exchange, (3) creating an open climate of participative creativity, (4) establishing an intent to change by forecasting the benefits, (5) translating the desire to change into action, (6) accepting local reinvention of the innovation as integral to the process, and (7) facilitating adoption by the opinion leaders. Ideally, external change agents are respectable, are similar to social system members, have technical expertise, and have competence and credibility. They work through opinion leaders and in some ways take some of the heat by absorbing the uncertainty and risk in the adoption process.

The notion of employees as internal change agents is nearly ubiquitous in every new job description. For many reasons, this role of change agent is rarely successful for internal employees. A better role for employees in the diffusion process is as facilitators of change, creating a safe place for risk-taking, creativity, and innovation, promoting open exchange and participation, and maintaining a customer-focused, vision-driven view of change. The role of early adopter is certainly a relatively safe position to take as long as adopted innovations are sound. If an employee occupies the role of opinion leader, this also may be satisfactory in terms of future security and status within the group.

Even though change agents serve a very important role in group survival, internal change agents tend to alienate the majority by regularly differentiating themselves from the group norm. This is why change agency is best accomplished through external agents who pass muster for their expertise and similarity to the organizational members and yet are not vested long term in the social system.

Organizational characteristics, which are frequently under the influence of management, have certain variables correlated with adoption of innovations. Positive correlations are decentralization, informality, interconnectedness, organizational slack (lessened financial control), and larger size, as well as a positive attitude toward change and risk tolerance among individual leaders and executives. Leader-executive roles in adoption of innovations include agenda setting, matching of opportunities with the organizational strengths, reinventing, clarifying, focusing, offering incentives, team-based performance profiling, and finally, routinizing of the change management process.

Interdisciplinary Clinical Work Teams

Classic sociotechnical systems design recommends joint optimization of the technical and social subsystems for work design. The most common method of joint optimization has been the implementation of self-directed, semiautonomous work teams in the relevant domain. The concept of patient-focused care was developed as an extension of self-directed work teams, as interdisciplinary workers with similar goals worked as a proximal unit to meet the needs of a defined group of patients with similar recurring problems. Multiskilled, cross-trained workers, optimal information sharing, and efficient work processes are the hallmarks of successful patient-focused care units.

Self-directed work teams require clear definition of their boundaries and scope of services in addition to clearly delineated authority and accountability. Precise descriptions of team goals and objectives along with team-based incentives and shared accountability are key elements of successful design.

There are several examples of successful work team applications in health care (Manion, Lorimer, & Leander, 1996). Unfortunately, physicians are frequently not included in the health care work team. Physician psyches have been characterized as fiercely independent, akin to those of cats and eagles, and physician culture as either masochistic or nonexistent.

In reality, physician social linkages are strong, albeit not always harmonious. The economic environment of the cottage industry, with small competing practices, has driven feelings of rivalry among physicians providing similar services. However, for the successful practice of medicine, intense, effective, and ongoing relationships are necessary, and most physicians recognize this.

Inclusion of physicians in self-directed work teams is of paramount importance, whether these are unit-based functional care delivery teams or performance improvement task forces. The synergy obtained from combining physicians, nurses, therapists, clinical service (laboratory, pharmacy, imaging) personnel, and facilities support staff is momentous, especially with regard to the work these teams can do in identifying performance gaps, understanding work processes, and adopting and diffusing innovations.

For the purposes of medical management, self-directed work teams have many advantages. An appropriately aligned and empowered work team offers the social structure to facilitate adoption of innovations, cost effectiveness, patient satisfaction, and outcomes management. Workflow may become more efficient and robust as technical requirements are matched more closely with the social setting of work team members. Teams have more flexibility and autonomy to handle individual patient needs in a timely manner. Implementation of changes can occur more quickly within the work team, as well as acceptance and modification of those changes.

Medical management may best be deployed through the self-directed work team and coordinated care approach. The alternative is a medical review model, in which an independent, detached critic passes judgment on the actions of individual providers, with no real sense of the ultimate outcome for the patient. All of the efforts are spent denying particular interventions and very little effort is expended on what the outcome needs to be and how to get there.

Clinical effectiveness projects may readily be conducted through established or ad hoc work teams. The process starts with vision alignment around a common set of goals, objectives, expectations, and boundaries. Team members *sign up* on patient care issues they care deeply about. A performance gap is established, or alternatively, a new opportunity is so enticing that the call to action is apparent to all.

Team members are identified, typically by self-selection or by coworker designation. Organizational research has identified the ideal size of the workgroup for decisive action as five to seven members. A group larger than that tends to exchange information rather than take action. A group smaller than that may be too limited in its view or perceived of as an imposing clique. If the body of work deliberation is more than a group of five to seven can deal with, smaller work teams, each with its own defined boundaries, can be initiated.

Root cause analysis through process analysis technique, along with drill-down data support at transaction-level detail, fosters the next phase. The work team will begin the process of discovery, explaining the performance gap and identifying opportunities for process changes that may create improvement. A pilot study at the institution frequently serves to bolster efforts and justify subsequent widespread changes.

The medical management work team then suggests several workflow modifications as standardized approaches to certain critical decision points. Frequently, these modifications are encapsulated in a clinical guideline (decision points) or a pathway (workflow components).

Ongoing value improvement analysis is also integral to the process. Improvement in outcomes (quality, service, access) as well as cost benefit establishes the success of the work team's efforts and the medical management program in general. Profiling performance on a system, facility, service line, unit, or individual basis cultivates goal setting and target achievement as well as alignment among all relevant parties who affect the improvement process.

The facilitator's role in clinical effectiveness work teams is also very helpful in focusing groups on the opportunities and value to be derived from the team's efforts. Nominal group technique is frequently used to generate creative solutions to problems, with decision making staged into discrete steps to prevent premature evaluation or group dynamics that may block idea generation. The Delphi technique polls domain experts anonymously for the purpose of idea generation for problem solution. Facilitators can help overcome group divisiveness and align team members' common ground. An atmosphere of diversity arising from multiple viewpoints is beneficial, and a good facilitator can stimulate this culture.

Project Management

Project management of clinical effectiveness and performance improvement projects is of substantial assistance in successful initiatives. Health care processes frequently require complex scheduling and resource coordination. Clinical effectiveness and performance improvement projects are typically intricate, involving several functions and departments. Project management is a methodology to chronicle mutual dependence and assign accountability for project completion through scheduling of resources and reminders.

Tools such as Gantt charts, which show tasks on the left side (y axis) and units of time on the bottom (x axis), enable visualization of the proposed project completion timeline and are integral to most project management software packages. However, the Gantt chart fails to show interdependencies between tasks or to convey information about potential bottlenecks or resource constraints.

Another tool used by project management software is the PERT chart (Program Evaluation and Review Technique). It graphically portrays the relationships among a multiplicity of specific tasks as well as the constraints. The PERT chart reveals the time estimate for each interdependency in a network of sequential and simultaneous tasks; a series of arrows and circle nodes define the relationships in the network. From this analysis, tasks can be properly sequenced for maximum throughput.

Project management software can also track project status, link to e-mail for reminders and updates, account for budgets and expenditures, and elucidate variances from expectations.

Clinical Measurement and Quantitative Analysis

The importance of objective data analysis in the accomplishment of medical management cannot be overemphasized. True appraisal of performance in a specified area drives the desire to improve. Information about cost, outcomes, and intermediate work process steps removes subjective and political appraisals of effectiveness.

Infrastructure Requirements. Medical management has several infrastructure requirements for successful application. The most important functions are information technology, decision support, data analysis and statistical findings, work team facilitation, and project management.

Information technology plays a key role in the data collection, analysis, and presentation process. Decision support databases must be modeled and maintained. Data must be transformed and interfaced from transaction legacy systems to the data warehouse. Individual workstations must be maintained and network connections, including Internet connectivity, must be sustained and high performing. Applications to analyze and present data must be available to and, ideally, used by frontline work team members (data farmers and tourists), not just backroom data analysts (data explorers).

Medical management is such an information-intensive endeavor that clinical measurement and quantitative analysis support are critical functions. Issues of severity in a patient population and unintended bias that confounds results are weighty matters when identifying performance gaps and potential causes. Statistical support is crucial, as many of these manipulations and determinations are beyond the capabilities and permissible time expenditures of work team members. Statisticians can work closely on project analysis and iterative development with work team members, adding value and understanding to the information and its presentation to others.

Another significant issue in clinical measurement is making *apples-to-apples* comparisons of data from multiple sources. Standardization of data element definitions, especially with regard to standard cost methodologies, is important when comparing or benchmarking. Often this is a time-consuming and challenging task, as organizational members must agree on a certain standard and give up their flexibility and latitude to a degree.

Comparative benchmarking is extremely enlightening about the level of work process and decision-making performance and can be a key motivator for change. Advanced statistical analysis is necessary for valid results when making comparisons. Furthermore, very large databases of coded data (from UB92 hospital discharge forms) may not give the clinical detail required to understand the root causes of performance gaps. Supplemental data from abstracted medical records may greatly assist a successful project.

The value of abstracted data may be weighed against its significant costs. Also, the consistency of the abstracted data element and, to an extent, interrater reliability may be relevant issues that require statistical interpretation.

These issues are exemplified in a clinical effectiveness project on stroke, using a very large database and supplemental abstracted data. In stroke, it is important that timely thrombolytic therapy be delivered to a select group of patients with discrete indications (stroke symptoms that appeared within the last three hours and a CT scan consistent with stroke) who have none of the significant contraindications (history of bleeding, coagulopathy, or recent surgery). Coded data frequently do not encompass the clinical granularity required to analyze whether the thrombolytics were delivered in a timely manner and to the right patients (indications) and were withheld for those who were not right (contraindications). Abstracted data may reveal such things as door-to-drug time in minutes and the presence or absence of discrete clinical issues (medical history, results of laboratory or imaging tests, and so forth) and can be of great value in clinical effectiveness projects.

The blending of abstracted data with coded data in very large databases has significant implications for interpretation and extrapolation. Abstracting medical records is expensive ($1 per data element), and usually only a limited sample of the database population is taken.

Analytical Techniques. For data analysis of clinical effectiveness or performance improvement projects to proceed, there are several considerations: (1) standardization of data elements (meanings and definitions), (2) severity determination (adjustment or stratification), (3) data element collection, storage, and quality control (very large administrative databases, abstracted medical records), and (4) use of surveys for patient-derived scales (functional status, satisfaction).

Standardizing meanings and definitions of data elements among diverse clinicians and medical staff is a daunting task, but it is necessary to guarantee apples-to-apples comparisons. For example, even in coded ICD-9 elements, there is no precise standardization of an element such as anemia. Is it hemoglobin or hematocrit? What is the precise threshold for normal values? Hemoglobin 14? Hemoglobin 15? Is the determination of anemia reflective of a change or an absolute value? What about agreement on the definitions of various types of anemia: Iron deficiency? Chronic disease? Macrocytic? It is quite helpful if clinicians at a given institution agree on the discrete elements and their definitions.

Issues arise over the choice of data elements themselves. Despite the tendency for staff to want to have every conceivable clinically relevant condition or nuance represented in the database, it is better to reduce the choices to those data elements that *make a difference* or are absolutely critical when evaluating dependencies among variables. At times various national organizations have popularized data repositories and promulgated de facto standard lexicons for their various domains that must be adhered to by all participants.

Severity determination is also highly relevant for physicians. Indeed, differences like "my patients are sicker" are usually overestimated by physicians. However, differences in populations can accrue through adverse selection, especially when a delivery system has a center of excellent reputation and attracts the toughest cases. Case mix and age-sex adjustments may explain to some degree the risk variation in populations. Most severity systems have attempted to quantify risks of short-term outcomes for an episode of care involving hospitalization. The severity measures may identify hard and true medical outcomes such as mortality, complications, or readmissions and expected resource use. Most severity systems use standard coded data elements (ICD-9) from hospital discharge forms. Some severity systems use a probability range (0 to 1), others use integer score (0 to 60), and yet others a scoring class (0 to 4). Many systems have been vigorously tested for their reliability, precision, and reproducibility. In addition, many studies have favorably reported on the validity or believability of the results when the severity system in question has been used in specific clinical situations.

Data quality control, collection, and storage are all important issues to address in clinical effectiveness studies. There is always a trade-off between extra data element collection for clinical credibility and the expense of abstracting data manually. A systematic evaluation of each of the proposed data elements is recommended to study the feasibility of collection and the reliability and accuracy of the data sources. Periodic audits to examine data quality are especially helpful, as interventions may be engineered at data entry to improve the quality of data collected. Accuracy of coding from hospital discharge forms may need to be addressed, as well as completeness and exactness of chart entries when abstracting elements from the medical record. Interrater reliability in reference to human coders or abstractors occurs as a consequence of individual training and background and to a certain degree as a result of any pressures the subject is working under that affect completeness or timing. Several methods exist to measure or audit interrater reliability, and interventions may be employed to lessen the variability, such as feedback and training on certain problematic data element interpretations or increased standardization of data element definitions at entry.

Finally, patient-derived scales, from surveys of functional status and satisfaction in particular, are increasingly valued as important adjuncts to clinical effectiveness projects. The coded, clinically relevant quality or medical content–based outcomes are limited in their richness. Mortality, readmissions, some complications, and few success measures can be appreciated in coded administrative databases. The ability to discern valid and reliable patient satisfaction and functional status determinations as medically relevant outcomes of care can be very valuable. Satisfaction scores are worthy in that they reflect service quality in health care delivery as much as the discrete medical outcome. Functional status and health-related quality of life scores allow assessment of the impact of sickness or a medical intervention on the basic health-related functions of life. A commonly used health status questionnaire is Short Form 36 (SF-36), which addresses aspects of mental and physical functioning, including specific appraisals of emotional role, physical role, bodily pain, general health, vitality, and social functioning.

Physicians, especially, appreciate the simultaneous linkage of utilization and cost-reduction efforts with medical outcomes such as patient satisfaction and functional status. Systems are available that allow integration of these patient-derived results with transaction detailed systems, enabling linkage of discrete utilization interventions with the outcomes of patient satisfaction and health-related quality of life.

Benchmarking

Comparative benchmarking may have great impact on both the establishment of the performance gap and the psychological impact of change and approach to problem solving at the organization. Even though internal benchmarking is anonymous, it is inherently adversarial, as performers are competitively compared with one another in terms of critical delivery outcomes or process measures. Tabular physician profiling and four-quadrant bubble graphing are frequent methods of portraying how internal performers stack up against one another (see addendum). The poorer performing providers realize they must change practices to match the high performers. The focus tends to be on individual efforts to improve decision making to overcome the deficit. Higher performers may have no incentive to further improve as they rest comfortably on their past performance. Typically, the performance gap is somewhat meager. Major special cause variations due to system deficiencies in care delivery may be ignored.

External comparative benchmarking addresses many of the issues raised with internal benchmarking. Undoubtedly, however, external benchmarking entails a greater expense and the task of standardizing data element definitions, especially for standard cost comparisons.

External benchmarking generally establishes a much larger performance gap, because the *best practice* from a larger population is identified. System deficiencies in care delivery may be uncovered, and efforts may be focused on how to improve the system in addition to improving individual performance. This frequently promotes a collaborative approach within the organization to optimize, even foolproof, system processes.

Benchmarking systems may present summary information or transaction-level detail of coded or abstracted data. Greater detail enables a greater ability to drill into discrete, executable process improvements or even decision points in a process of care. For example, detail that allows an internist to know the average numbers for a specific line item, such as chest X rays for simple pneumonia, gives that physician the knowledge and the incentive to alter his or her ordering of that particular item to match the ordering of the perceived best performer. Physicians especially value multidimensional studies that address how quality outcomes are either improved or at least held steady as utilization and costs are lowered. Transaction-level detail is frequently an important aspect of the benchmarking system. Likewise, standardization of cost methodology adds meaning, as actual charges contain an inherent and typically arbitrary inflation factor and are not trusted by physicians. Severity determination is also important to physicians, especially when comparing outcomes across institutions and locations where adverse selection or differing standards of care may exist. The addendum illustrates opportunity assessment, drill-down analysis, and physician profiling with a comparative benchmarking system.

Communication and Innovation

The potency of a medical management program in changing practices depends on communication among the physicians, workers, and administrators in the organization as well as connectedness to external best practices.

An organized approach to communication and clinical leadership is well worth the effort because it smooths the way for medical management and clinical effectiveness projects.

In general, and in physician culture specifically, there is a great liability in the *exalted leader* approach. It is impractical to count on the probability that a single charismatic figure will be available who has enough domain expertise and respect in every relevant constituency. Physicians fit the diffusion of innovations model quite well in that their social system selects and employs multiple opinion leaders, mostly informal, to guide the process of change. For the administrator responsible for medical management or those interested in championing such an effort, it is wise to understand the necessity of working with and through the selected opinion leaders in a social system. The role of the administrator in such situations should be to clarify the performance gap, envision, facilitate communication, contribute resources for exploration, and support established or rising opinion leaders.

A key element is the establishment of a common vision that inspires all of the relevant participants. They must possess a certain amount of trust in the organization in order to accept a vision that mutually benefits all the major parties. This trust-building and vision alignment takes time and consistency of intent and frequently requires the ability to link common initiatives when feasible to align constituents even more tightly.

A focus on external performance is frequently beneficial from an internal team building and collaboration perspective. Internal focus tends to establish a status quo and then to cause political action that ingratiates the representatives of the status quo in comfortable positions of power and status. Worker creativity and innovation may even be stifled as opponents of the status quo. An external focus first identifies how the internal system measures up to the best performer in a larger field. True collaboration to make the system better, through creativity and innovation from frontline workers, typically results.

External change agents may be of great benefit in this setting. Of course, as discussed earlier, they must be respectable, credible, relevant, and homophilous (possessing the same qualities as members) to the unique social system. These change agents may bring the external perspective necessary to stretch the vision of the organization, but at the same time they must possess a certain humility and respect for the internal social system and processes as they exist. The key to success as an external change agent is to identify and work with the opinion leaders to introduce, reinvent, and establish innovations. For administrators, enhancing a fertile management culture for change, creativity, and innovation should be the goal.

External change agents are vested only in the positive trajectory of the organization, not in their own future as an organizational member. This enables them to be somewhat risk tolerant and to withstand political skirmishes.

Conclusion

Information-driven medical management for performance improvement is no small undertaking. Value-based approaches are the best way to understand and provide incentives for improvement in health care delivery processes. Attention to the social, interpersonal, and communication channels of the delivery system in question is critically important.

Critical factors for successful information-driven medical management include effective information technology infrastructure, clinical measurement and quantitative analysis support, project management, physician support alliances, coordination of care, and decision support systems. A culture that promotes participation, open communication, and facilitation of self-directed work teams is vitally important. Consideration of the techniques in successful data analysis, such as data standardization, severity determination, data quality, comparative benchmarking, and patient-derived scales, is important.

Finally, interchange among physicians, workers, and administration staff greatly enhances the speed and success of medical management programs. Establishment of a common trustworthy and acceptable vision, use of external change agents, and a focus on external comparisons promotes nonthreatening collaboration and circum-spection, enhancing internal change, creativity, and innovation.

Addendum: Examples of Data

Opportunity Assessment:
DRG 127—Heart Failure and Shock

The opportunity assessment in Figure 6.3 reveals sixteen DRGs with cost-savings opportunities for a client health system. For each DRG, the average length of stay (ALOS) and average direct costs (laboratory, pharmacy, imaging, supplies) are com-pared with the benchmark. Variance per discharge is calculated, as is the potential cost opportunity for each DRG in calendar year 1997. The benchmark group may reflect mean, median, and a certain percentile (or the best practice) identified in the study group.

DRG 127 (heart failure and shock) reveals a client ALOS of 5.76 and average direct cost of $3,286 compared with the bench-mark values of 4.62 and $2,397, respectively. This reveals a vari-ance per discharge of $889 and a cost opportunity on 567 patients for 1997 of $504,063, if performance at the client health system could match the benchmark.

The remaining question is where the opportunities reside. Pharmacy, laboratory, and imaging and supply cost detail with benchmarks could reveal the answer.

External Comparative Benchmarking:
Cost Variance Report with Physician Detail

Physician specific costs are portrayed for DRG 127, heart failure and shock (Figure 6.4). Note that PMI represents patient mix index (an HBSI™ methodology) that uses case-mix, severity-adjusted data to take into account the illness burden among groups of patients that are being compared. It is a measure of the expected relative intensity for the group of patients under study.

Figure 6.3. Opportunity Assessment. HBSI EXPLORE™ Clinical Benchmarking System. Average Direct Costs and Lengths of Stay by DRG, January 1, 1997 to December 31, 1997.

DRG	Client Patient Count	Benchmark Patient Count	Client ALOS	Benchmark ALOS	Client Average Direct Costs	Benchmark Direct Costs	Direct Costs Variance per DC	Potential Cost Opportunity
373	3,105	14,959	1.76	1.86	$1,352	$1,102	$ 250	$ 776,250
430	670	3,730	7.22	7.03	$2,401	$2,202	$ 199	$ 133,330
371	821	3,071	3.02	3.13	$2,602	$1,820	$ 782	$ 642,022
89	678	2,484	6.55	5.34	$3,493	$2,539	$ 954	$ 646,812
88	395	2,359	6.44	4.57	$2,456	$2,038	$ 418	$ 165,110
372	412	2,793	2.33	2.35	$2,234	$1,303	$ 931	$ 383,572
127	567	2,355	5.76	4.62	$3,286	$2,397	$ 889	$ 504,063
359	256	1,972	2.34	2.29	$2,213	$1,930	$ 283	$ 72,448
374	341	1,637	2.01	2.09	$2,123	$1,691	$ 432	$ 147,312
14	304	1,475	7.58	5.18	$3,977	$3,374	$ 603	$ 183,312
370	198	1,805	3.65	3.66	$3,432	$2,092	$ 1,340	$ 265,320
124	315	1,155	3.23	3.57	$3,467	$2,740	$ 727	$ 229,005
209	178	1,173	4.58	4.51	$6,312	$5,544	$ 768	$ 136,704
121	165	1,032	4.82	6.07	$5,392	$3,923	$ 1,469	$ 242,385
122	186	657	3.42	4.03	$4,121	$3,197	$ 924	$ 171,864
79	134	749	8.39	7.16	$4,754	$3,476	$ 1,278	$ 171,252
	8,725	43,406						$4,870,761

Source: HBSI EXPLORE™ with permission.

Figure 6.4. Cost Variance Report.

Selection Criteria

Hospital ID: [ ]

GROUPED BY:	Service Line
SUBGROUPED BY:	A-DRG, Attend Phys ID
NORM:	

Grouping	Total Cases	PMI	Avg Cost/ PMI	Avg Cost Var/ PMI	Avg LOS/ PMI	Avg PDay Var/ PMI
CARDIOLOGY	1,973	1.26	3,626	−558	2.9	−.11
127 Heart Failure & Shock	408	0.93	3,805	−169	5.1	.08
1680	41	0.91	3,623	−357	5.3	.32
1579	34	0.93	3,036	−941	4.2	−.85
0452	30	0.90	2,743	−1,238	3.7	−1.18
1250	23	0.94	5,455	1,484	8.4	3.41
0553	15	0.89	3,885	−86	5.2	.31
1346	15	1.07	4,873	937	4.8	.06
1379	15	0.74	3,129	−885	5.1	−.02
0427	13	0.83	3,437	−557	4.8	−.27
0177	12	0.90	4,254	275	7.6	2.73
0142	11	1.05	3,575	−398	4.0	−1.05
1356	11	1.07	3,452	−499	4.6	−.27
0145	11	0.83	3,487	−511	4.6	−.51
1890	10	1.02	6,263	2,316	7.3	2.42
0201	8	0.84	4,198	215	5.5	.44
0589	8	0.82	3,584	−438	4.7	−.38
0660	8	0.82	3,036	−960	4.7	−.35
0376	8	1.04	2,890	−1,083	3.6	−1.45
0204	7	0.87	4,556	557	5.3	.17
0432	7	0.89	3,758	−227	6.4	1.32
0175	6	0.94	3,496	−476	3.4	−1.68
0470	6	0.91	3,958	−29	4.6	−.48
0130	5	0.89	3,704	−268	5.2	.12
0379	5	0.78	3,955	−37	6.2	1.06
0388	5	0.93	2,797	−1,192	4.3	−.75
0132	5	0.96	3,291	−681	3.3	−1.73
0178	4	0.77	2,744	−1,253	3.6	−1.54
1506	4	0.90	4,539	568	6.4	1.29
0783	4	1.37	3,562	−351	3.5	−1.17
0350	4	0.64	2,761	−1,336	3.5	−1.69
0174	3	0.94	3,343	−629	4.6	−.43
0211	3	0.94	3,138	−834	4.6	−.43
0423	3	0.76	2,228	−1,778	3.5	−1.59
1340	3	0.81	4,337	367	3.7	−1.39

Average Department Costs per PMI									
Pharm		Image		Lab		Supply		Other	
Costs	Cost Var	Costs	Cost Var	Costs	Cost Var	Costs	Cost Var	Costs	Cost Var
193	24	100	−46	143	−28	409	−273	2,781	−235
307	110	114	−7	223	−52	193	−19	2,968	−201
388	194	109	−13	201	−75	113	−98	2,811	−367
227	30	57	−64	242	−34	128	−84	2,383	−789
147	−47	103	−20	196	−78	107	−107	2,190	−985
457	258	141	20	350	75	222	9	4,286	1,122
353	161	191	67	145	−129	184	−29	3,013	−157
435	217	116	−1	234	−37	466	245	3,623	513
148	−13	63	−67	136	−141	141	−62	2,641	−603
224	46	75	−50	184	−93	145	−61	2,809	−400
478	284	160	36	185	−89	117	−98	3,314	143
223	13	166	48	178	−98	155	−59	2,853	−302
278	63	79	−38	197	−76	198	−21	2,700	−427
248	69	40	−85	117	−160	216	9	2,866	−344
370	160	397	278	308	35	433	215	4,756	1,627
473	295	160	37	304	28	131	−75	3,129	−70
351	172	42	−86	167	−111	196	−11	2,828	−401
279	104	109	−16	168	−109	132	−74	2,349	−864
219	9	128	10	321	45	152	−62	2,069	−1,086
332	146	129	5	279	2	260	52	3,555	352
368	179	67	−55	216	−60	136	−73	2,972	−217
295	100	58	−62	163	−113	122	−88	2,858	−314
462	271	56	−66	136	−141	261	51	3,043	−144
368	181	43	−78	183	−93	172	−36	2,939	−242
152	−15	123	−4	110	−166	96	−107	3,474	255
278	83	35	−87	193	−84	45	−166	2,247	−939
325	126	39	−81	206	−70	210	−1	2,512	−656
234	68	102	−25	106	−170	120	−83	2,183	−1,042
320	131	240	119	281	6	210	2	3,488	310
332	86	202	90	305	35	178	−52	2,545	−510
135	−4	77	−66	154	−129	147	−53	2,248	−1,084
245	50	26	−94	286	10	359	149	2,428	−744
111	−83	49	−71	245	−31	112	−98	2,622	−550
103	−60	42	−87	187	−89	103	−100	1,793	−1,442
263	91	353	229	557	283	301	97	2,864	−333

Excludes transfers and outliers and cases where no available norm.
Source: HBSI EXPLORE™ with permission. Copyright 1996 HBS International, Inc.

Notice the cost variances for DRG 127, heart and failure shock. The pharmacy cost variance is $110, revealing an opportunity, and imaging, radiology, and supply costs are actually better than the external benchmark.

Notice the significant variation among physicians in the areas of pharmacy, laboratory, and imaging, as well as ALOS and average cost per PMI. Physician 1250 has an average cost/PMI of $5,455 (cost variance from benchmark $1,484), ALOS/PMI of 8.4 days (benchmark 3.41), pharmacy costs of $475 (variance from benchmark $258), imaging cost of $141 (variance $20), and lab cost of $350 (variance $75), thus revealing plenty of opportunities with this physician.

System-based interventions, such as guidelines for utilization, that affect decision points in order entry may result in the desired improvements.

Physician Profiling: Bubble Graph—LOS/Cost Variance

Figure 6.5 uses the four-quadrant bubble graph technique to emphasize physician performance. By convention, opportunities are presented in the upper outer quadrant, as in this case, high cost/high LOS for DRG 127, heart failure and shock.

The norm for DRG 127 is portrayed at the intersection of the x- and y-axis at 0.0. The x-axis represents average cost variance, and the y-axis, patient day LOS variance. Most of the physicians portrayed have efficient LOS, and costs are better than the norm. Physicians C and D have opportunities for improvement; physician C has opportunities for improvement in both cost and LOS.

Physician Profiling

Figure 6.6 represents a tabular physician profiling report for DRG 127, heart failure and shock. The physician portrayed may compare his or her performance with several peer groups within the health

**Figure 6.5. Bubble Graph Report. LOS/Cost Variance
A-DRG 127—Heart Failure and Shock,
Top Volume Physicians Client Hospital.**

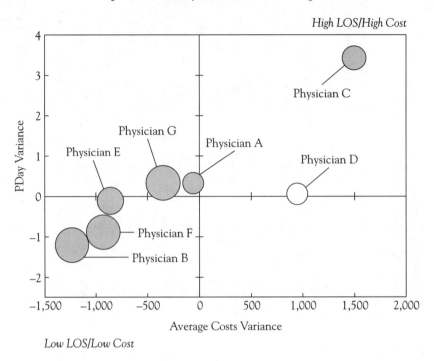

Source: HBSI EXPLORE™ with permission.

system (other physicians in the department, all physicians, and internists only) and externally with hospitals A, B, D, E, and a national peer group.

Notice there are comparisons for lab, imaging, drugs, and direct costs, as well as LOS and mortality. The PMI (patient mix index) and average age of the physician's patients are comparable also.

This physician has less illness burden in his or her population than the norm, and compares quite favorably in all groups with costs, including direct, lab, pharmacy, and imaging. LOS is favorably comparable with most groups, and mortality is exemplary.

Figure 6.6. Physician Profiling Report.

Discharge Period: Between 01-Jan-1997 and 31-Dec-1997
Physician Role: ATD

Hospital:
Physician:
ADRG Code: 127–Heart Failure & Shock

Patient Type: Inpatients
Between Ages 0 and 99

	Physician	Other	Hospital	Internal Medicine	HOSP A	HOSP B	HOSP D	HOSP E	Peer Group
Total Patients	20	219	239	87	219	258	938	125	1779
Average Age	70.80	75.76	75.35	73.37	74.14	71.53	73.49	78.74	73.90
Average LOS	5.05	5.57	5.53	5.79	5.12	5.05	4.85	4.11	4.95
Average Total Costs	$3,327	$3,990	$3,935	$4,502	$5,031	$4,405	$4,258	$5,140	$4,393
Average Lab Units	21.90	27.08	26.64	32.14	58.09	27.90	34.39	24.94	34.66
Average Lab Costs	$254	$312	$307	$384	$408	$259	$265	$338	$293
Average Image Units	1.95	2.58	2.52	2.63	2.55	2.86	4.23	2.30	3.46
Average Image Costs	$56	$83	$81	$96	$84	$96	$152	$69	$120
Average Drug Units	136.35	149.96	148.82	166.80	119.62	126.66	143.11	80.66	134.21
Average Drug Costs	$166	$253	$246	$282	$265	$166	$299	$167	$259
Average Direct Costs	$1,722	$2,143	$2,108	$2,442	$2,755	$2,689	$2,604	$2,608	$2,569
Patient Mix Index (PMI)	0.92	1.12	1.10	1.17	1.05	0.92	0.96	0.89	0.98
Percent (%) Mortality	0	5.02%	4.60%	8.05%	6.85%	4.65%	3.30%	7.20%	4.38%

*Date Ranges: HOSP A Jan 1996–Dec 1996, HOSP B Jan 1996–Dec 1996, HOSP D Jan 1996–Dec 1996, HOSP E Jan 1996–Dec 1996
HBSI Outliers: IL

PMI calculations are based only on HBSI Inlier data.
HBSI Physician Profiling Report 2.0.320 Monday, October 13, 1997 10:25 PM

CONFIDENTIAL, PEER REVIEW DATA
Copyright: 1997

Source: HBSI EXPLORE™ with permission.

Part Two

Issues in Information Management

Part Two presents issues in the practical use of information management to support improvement in health care performance. Case studies that illustrate the complexity of the integration and application of health care information are explored.

Chapter Seven

Legal Issues in Management of Health Care Data

Patricia Driscoll

A clinically integrated approach to data
management for the purpose of improving the
quality, effectiveness, and outcomes of care requires
that providers share patient information—
including very personal clinical information—to a
far greater degree than has previously been the
norm. Many uses for publicly valuable, quality data
have emerged, but with them comes increased
responsibility. This chapter discusses the nature of
health care information, emerging trends in
legislation to protect privacy, and issues in
developing data policy.

The increased emphasis upon value-based health care purchasing decisions has fueled efforts to produce, share, and evaluate data purporting to address the components of health care value. The changing health care market, regulatory reform, and the trend toward increased consumer involvement in health care purchasing decisions have stimulated the release of information to the public about quality of care and outcomes.

The quality-performance-value nexus operates through data generation, dissemination, and publication. Although health care organizations have a responsibility to provide information about quality, they have an equal responsibility not to publish or release certain types of patient data. The duty of the clinical knowledge worker to protect the confidentiality and privacy of the patient must be met even as the worker aggregates information to improve care. The emphasis on data coupled with legal ambiguity regarding privacy requirements has given rise to a host of legal concerns. However, the legal issues should not pose an insurmountable barrier to effective information management. Instead, the prudent health care provider and knowledge worker will embrace data technology and the information it can provide, yet also insist on optimum levels of privacy and security.

An individual's health care record contains private information relating to such things as family history, genetic testing, previous diseases and their treatment outcomes, substance use, sexual orientation, and sexually transmitted diseases, as well as subjective assessments regarding the person's demeanor, mental state, and character. Secondary users of this type of information, such as employers, insurance companies, educational institutions, or governmental agencies, could exploit it to influence decisions about an individual's access to credit, admission to educational institutions, ability to obtain insurance, and ability to secure and maintain employment (Electronic Frontier Foundation, 1993).

Information inaccuracies or improper disclosure can have catastrophic personal, professional, and financial results, which may be irreversible. Therefore, it is not surprising that attention to the confidentiality and security of patient information has led to a proliferation of legal strictures on access to health care data at the same time that demand for more and better information about care quality and effectiveness is heightened.

Legal Confidentiality Requirements

While engaged in the process of finding and processing health care information, the clinical knowledge worker must recognize the inherent tension between sharing patient information to facilitate the integrated delivery of care and the assessment of the quality and outcomes of that care and complying with legal confidentiality requirements. The complexity of legal confidentiality requirements and the difficulty of achieving full compliance with them is due in large part to the fact that the law has generally lagged behind advances in health information technology. Much of the statutory framework of the law was developed in an era of paper records and an absence of data sharing.

Legal requirements concerning the confidentiality of patient information are found in the Constitution of the United States and the constitutions of the various states, in federal and state statutes and regulations (including the Medicare conditions of participation), and in the common law (that body of law derived from judicial decisions and precedents). The Supreme Court has recognized a limited constitutional right to information privacy, but the rulings in cases germane to this issue have been extremely narrow in scope. Virtually all the cases dealing with information privacy that the Court has ruled on involve dissemination of information by a branch of government. Because most of the health data activities are taking place in private, nongovernmental entities, the constitutional right to privacy will probably afford little protection for the type of breaches that opponents to automation fear.

Most states have recognized a private right of action (right to sue) for invasion of privacy. The common law concept of privacy most applicable to health care providers and those involved in quality management is the right of the individual to "be let alone" and protected from the public disclosure of private facts. Public disclosure of private facts applies to the publication (sharing with third parties) of private information about an individual without consent, even when the facts are true and therefore not subject to an action for libel or slander. Damage awards have been upheld by the courts in cases involving the public disclosure of photographs or films of individuals even though these materials were used for instructional purposes. For a person to prevail in a suit for invasion of privacy, he or she must show that the disclosure has been made public; the facts disclosed were private facts, not public ones; and the matter made public was something that would be offensive or objectionable to a reasonable person of ordinary sensibilities.

Some states (for example, California, Maryland, Minnesota, Montana, Rhode Island, Washington, and Wisconsin) also impose confidentiality requirements through general health information confidentiality statutes. However, the more common state approach is to impose legal confidentiality requirements through regulatory requirements such as licensure. These confidentiality requirements may vary, depending on who records or maintains the patient information.

State laws thus form a patchwork of confidentiality requirements. For example, only twenty-eight states have legal provisions allowing patients to access their own medical records for information or accuracy.

Federal and state statutes and regulations impose strict confidentiality requirements for records containing certain very sensitive patient information, such as records of alcohol and drug abuse treatment (U.S. Code, vol. 42, sec. 290dd–2; Code of Federal Regulations, vol. 42, part 2), mental health records (see, for example, Iowa Code, Annotated, sec. 228.1), records containing HIV test results or information indicating an AIDS diagnosis (see, for example, Ohio Revised Code, sec. 301.243), and increasingly, information from genetic screening and testing results (see, for example, 1995 Oregon Laws, 680). These statutes generally permit disclosure of the protected information only pursuant to a specific consent or authorization or in accordance with a limited list of exceptions. Because penalties for violating these special confidentiality laws are generally greater than those for disclosing nonsensitive medical information, clinical knowledge workers should consider excluding this protected information or at least employing special security measures for it when using or pooling patient information in data repositories. Many of the sensitive health information confidentiality statutes also prohibit redisclosure of protected information by recipients to whom it is legally disclosed, unless redisclosure is authorized by a valid consent or other exception. Because the access of other providers (between physician and hospital and health plan) to protected information will generally constitute a redisclosure of the information, strict access controls will be necessary for all information of this type.

Because confidentiality requirements vary from state to state, the issue of which state's confidentiality law applies in a given case may arise. This is particularly true when dealing with health information networks and multistate locations of patients, providers, and data. The issue is complicated by the consolidation of the health care industry, the increased mobility of consumers, the proximity of providers and consumers to state lines, the use of e-mail and other electronic communication in daily business operations, and the emergence of telemedicine and the delivery of health care services over the Internet. The determination of which state's law to follow may depend on the location of the patient when care was delivered, the location of the provider making the medical record entries, and where the medical record is stored. These conflicts along with an absence of federal standards that define privacy and confidentiality requirements have led to a call for preemptive federal patient confidentiality legislation that would create a single national standard for patient confidentiality and would clarify health care providers' obligations and patients' rights regarding health care information.

Proposed Federal Regulations

The Health Insurance Portability and Accountability Act of 1996 (HIPAA) spells out broad guidelines for a new, strict national policy covering personally identifiable health care information. Instead of specifically mandating a comprehensive and national approach to privacy and confidentiality, HIPAA charged the secretary of Health and Human Services (HHS) with adopting standards on the use and misuse of personally identifiable health care data and standards to govern the security and safeguarding of data collected and processed electronically (Subtitle F, Administrative Simplification, U.S. *Code*, vol. 42, secs. 1301 et seq., part C, secs. 1171–1175). Pursuant to HIPAA, on September 11, 1997, the secretary delivered recommendations intended to assist Congress in drafting appropriate legislation (U.S. Department of Health and Human Services, 1997). None of the recommendations has yet been adopted into law, and it is important to remember that the exact form of any law enacted may be dramatically different from these initial recommendations. However, these recommendations provide guidance that prudent providers and payers can and should consider when developing policies and procedures for information systems and data handling.

The proposed national standard of confidentiality embodied in the secretary's recommendations was organized around five key principles: appropriate boundaries, security, consumer control, accountability, and public responsibility.

Boundaries

The recommendations state that an individual's health care information should be used only for health purposes, subject to a few carefully defined exceptions. In addition, the same duty of confidentiality applicable to those who provide health care should be imposed on those who pay for health care services and on any other entities that receive health information from them. The secretary recommended that federal legislation address the following four areas:

1. Provision of and payment for health care. Federal law should limit the ways that providers and payers can use identifiable health information, protect information used in research, and cover employers that render on-site health care or provide benefits. Congress should continue to examine hazards to pri-

vacy when nonproviders or payers hold health information, and should regulate appropriately.

2. Service organizations. Claims processors, pharmacy benefits managers, information systems and service vendors with access to data files, and any other service organizations should be subject to federal law and the same confidentiality restrictions as providers and payers. Agreements between a provider or payer and a service organization should contain an explicit commitment on the part of the service organization to avoid unauthorized use or distribution of health information. The agreement should also provide notice to the service organization that it will be subject to federal and state privacy laws. (Given this recommendation, it would be prudent to require confidentiality agreements between any two organizations that transfer data—even if they are both entities of the same network or parent company.)

3. Disclosure with authorization. If a patient authorizes disclosure to a third person, he or she should be able to enforce an agreement with that person about how the information may be used. Federal law may impose an enforceable contract between the patient and the recipient of the information.

4. Limited disclosure for national priorities. The law should provide exceptions to strict confidentiality requirements for the purposes of maintaining public health, oversight of the health care system, research, and law enforcement.

Security

Disclosure of identifiable information should be limited to the minimum necessary to accomplish the purpose of the disclosure. The use of identifiable information within an organization should be limited to the purposes for which the information was collected, and patient authorization should have to meet specific requirements.

Consumer Control

Significant new consumer rights are included in the recommendations. These rights are similar to consumer credit rights. For example, it is recommended that providers and payers be required to advise patients in writing of their information practices. Patients should be able to see their records, get copies of them, and propose corrections. In addition, providers and payers should maintain a history of disclosures, and patients should be able to access that history.

Accountability

The recommendations provide punishment for those who misuse personal health information as well as legal redress for the persons harmed by that information's misuse. Criminal penalties would be imposed for obtaining health information under false pretenses and for knowingly disclosing or using medical information in violation of the federal privacy law. Penalties would include the possibility of substantial fines and of imprisonment. Individuals whose rights under the law are violated would be permitted to bring an action for monetary damages and injunctive relief. Monetary damages are intended to provide compensation for injury sustained due to violation of a person's rights. Injunctive relief consists of a court order prohibiting a person or entity from doing some specified act or engaging in certain behavior. An injunction is considered a preventive and protective remedy aimed at stopping future acts as opposed to addressing past wrongs. In addition, recovery of attorney's fees and punitive damages would be available against persons who knowingly violate the law.

Public Responsibility

The recommendations specify that any national privacy act passed pursuant to these recommendations should allow disclosure of health information for major national priorities as long as this information is disclosed and used only for its identified public purpose. This provision has already been widely criticized as overly broad and therefore is likely to be modified.

Data Security Issues

Preserving the confidentiality of electronic health information requires proper system and data security. Inadequate security affects not only the appropriate use and disclosure of information but also the ability of authorized users to access the data and the accuracy and integrity of the information. It is impossible to control all security risks in managing electronic patient-related information. No security system or measures generally used today can withstand the efforts of a skilled computer expert determined to break into a system. Because perfect security may be extremely difficult to achieve, it is important to determine what level of security is legally required.

The current legal standard as well as the regulatory standard recommended by the secretary of HHS for data security is reasonable and appropriate administrative, technical, and physical safeguards to ensure the integrity and confidentiality of health information and to protect against reasonably anticipated threats and hazards to the security or integrity of the information and unauthorized uses or disclosure of the patient's data.

Determining what constitutes reasonable security measures requires balancing several factors, including the threat posed, the acceptable level of restriction on the users, the ability to maintain the chosen security approach, the ability to reliably administer the approach, the effectiveness of specific components of the approach, and the cost to the organization. The American Health Information Management Association recommends organizations consider the following factors in determining the reasonableness of security: the state of commercially available technology; the affordability of security technology; the likelihood of a security failure and the risk that a failure could be caused intentionally; the magnitude of the harm that could result if security fails, is inadequate, or is breached; the known and reasonably anticipated threats to security; the standards promulgated by nationally recognized standard-setting organizations and professional associations in the fields of health information, health care informatics, and computer security; and the legal requirements concerning accessibility of patient records. However, complicating organizations' compliance efforts is the fact that the threats and hazards that constitute reasonably anticipated security issues will evolve and change as technology develops, as more health information becomes available through electronic media, including the Internet, and as increasingly sophisticated technology presents new threats to security. Therefore policies and approaches to system and data security must be reviewed and appropriately updated to remain reasonable. HIPAA's directive to the secretary to review security standards as necessary and adapt them to the changing information technology environment in the context of minimizing the disruption and cost of compliance should provide guidance, when implemented, in this dynamic area.

The secretary's recommendations regarding security encompass taking measures that include employee education, clear and certain punishment for misuses of information, and technical controls on access to information within an organization. Significant evidence suggests that a substantial threat to information is the careless or deliberate misuse by those who have authorized access to it in their normal work activities and not outsiders who hack into the system (U.S. Department of Health and Human Services, n.d.). A recent study by the National Research Council Computer Science and Telecommunications Board identifies current best practices for protecting privacy and maintaining security in health care information systems (National Research Council, 1997). Another resource is the series of publications from the Computer-Based Patient Record Institutes (CPRI) that contain guidance on security policies for computer-based patient records.

West Virginia is implementing an electronic medical record system for fourteen health service sites in three counties. The

ARTEMIS (Advanced Research Testbed for Medical Informatics) project includes identifying and addressing privacy issues as a part of centralizing patient information. Using high-resolution, high-performance hardware, the ARTEMIS system will make patient charts available at the various locations via an intranet system—a closed, firewall-protected database accessible via the Internet. Results from this project should provide useful information on implementation as well as security.

Examples of security measures that can be implemented by organizations that generate, access, and use patient care information include

- Access protection
- User authentication
- Audit trails
- Training and education
- Physical security
- Organizational policies and procedures
- An organizational culture conducive to privacy protection
- Built-in computer hardware and software security
- Secure hardware
- Secure operating systems
- Secure application software
- Secure communication protocols and methods (Appavu, 1997)

Legislative Activity

Major legislation has been introduced in Congress and in most state legislatures in 1999 governing the collection, maintenance, and disclosure of individually identifiable health information. This activity appears to be the result of a confluence of several strong concerns. First, the public is reacting to the rapid and pervasive effects of the information revolution and the perceived excesses of managed care and is putting pressure on elected officials. Second, section 264 of HIPAA mandated that the secretary of HHS promulgate regulations on medical privacy if Congress failed to enact legislation by August 21, 1999. Although several bills were introduced, Congress failed to pass a law by the deadline and the Department of HHS is preparing the rules for February 2000 issuance. A law passed by Congress would carry more weight than regulations issued by HHS. However, Congress can extend the deadline imposed by HIPPA or enact legislation prior to issuance of regulations. And finally, there is international pressure from the European Union (EU). The EU Data Protection Directive prohibits the transborder flow of data to countries that are not deemed to provide "adequate" protection of "personally identifiable" information. There is a perceived inequity between the security of health information, which contains highly personal data for which no federal protection exists, and the security of other personal information, such as credit reporting, banking, electronic mail, cable television, and video rental records, for which there are federal safeguards.

The Health Information Privacy Act of 1999 (the Condit-Waxman-Markey-Dingell bill in the House and the Bennett-Mack-Murkowski-Santorum bill in the Senate) was not passed; however, it provides some insight into the direction that Congress is likely to take on these complex issues. The proposed act is premised on three principles:

- Health information should not be used or disclosed without authorization or knowledge of the patient, except in narrow circumstances where there is an overriding public interest (such as protection of public health).
- Individuals should have fundamental rights regarding their health records, including the right to access, copy, and amend their records and the opportunity to seek special protection for especially sensitive records.

- Federal legislation should provide a *floor*, not a *ceiling*, allowing states and the secretary of HHS to establish additional protections (see www.house.gov).

The bill implements many of the recommendations of the secretary of HHS. Specifically, it

- Requires health care providers and payers to meet individuals' reasonable expectations of privacy regarding their health information.
- Prohibits the use or disclosure of health information without authorization or knowledge of patients, except in narrow circumstances. Using health information without authorization for purposes of marketing, employment, or insurance underwriting is specifically prohibited.
- Requires any authorization to be based on informed consent, not coerced through the withholding of health care treatment or payment.
- Provides essential rights, such as the right of individuals to view and amend their health information and seek special protections for sensitive information.
- Allows the use and disclosure of health information under appropriate circumstances for essential public interest purposes, including protection of public health, health research, health oversight, and law enforcement.
- Establishes a statutory floor for privacy protection that permits the secretary of HHS and the states to provide greater protection of health information.

Conclusion: Action Items for Clinical Knowledge Workers

The following checklist provides an information security and protection starting point for the clinical knowledge worker:

1. Make security and confidentiality of individually identifiable health information a priority in your organization, a priority demanding top-level executive participation.

2. Review the federal recommendations promulgated pursuant to HIPAA and the current legal requirements affecting electronic health data use and exchange in your jurisdiction. Keep in mind that HIPAA will supersede state law that is less stringent but will not preempt state law that is more protective.

3. Review state and federal program regulatory requirements for the storage, access, retrieval, security, and safeguarding of patient information in light of expanded electronic capabilities and in light of expected federal standards for patient access and review of such information.

4. Review corporate documents, medical staff bylaws, and any other relevant documentation to ensure that appropriate authorizations and internal standards have been established for the most efficient use of electronic and computerized patient records. This is necessary both to optimize usage of information systems and to meet the requirements of new legal standards and regulations. Medical staff need to be brought into the process to facilitate their buy-in.

5. Ensure that all vendors, suppliers, and service partners are brought into your security system through clearly drafted and detailed specifications of the requirements for confidentiality, security, and access limitation (including firewalls, encryption, authentication, and so forth).

6. Establish clearly articulated corporate or entity policies on the use and misuse of health care information, especially personally identifiable patient information.

7. Develop and provide training for all employees on the subject of privacy, and ensure that they have the tools and resources

needed to comply with confidentiality and security expectations.

8. Develop appropriate privacy policies and procedures to address new and evolving uses of electronic patient information, and ensure enforcement.

Chapter Eight

Adjusting for Severity

Clinical data exist today as an electronic by-
product of administrative functions. This chapter
discusses the limitations of administrative data for
measuring clinical outcomes and effectiveness, the
impact of vocabulary standardization on the
measurement of effectiveness and outcomes of care,
and the value of a team approach in selecting a
severity of illness system.

Although administrative, or claims-based, databases have been commonly used as a source for public reporting initiatives, providers must now search for more accurate and clinically robust data. They must determine whether variations in outcomes are due to clinical practice or the patients themselves. Adjustment of data for the risk or severity of illness of patients is an essential step in using the data and ultimately improving performance.

To understand the challenge of finding a rich source of clinical data, consider the objective of performance improvement: determining the clinical interventions and processes most effective for, beneficial to, and appreciated by typical patients and providers. A performance improvement study involves identifying unexplained variations in practice. It may consider barriers to care, whether financial, social, intellectual, or structural. It may encompass the diffusion of innovations as reflected in the environment, communications systems, and leadership. Outcome variables in a performance improvement study may include such subjective factors as symptom relief, functional status, satisfaction, quality of life, and social roles. A performance improvement study is fundamentally patient centered. Its results are pragmatic, generalizable, and have policy implications.

The Search for Severity Adjustment

Severity may be defined in physiological parameters with quantifiable biological factors. It may be defined functionally, in terms of an individual's ability to carry out daily activities. An additional and emerging dimension of severity is the illness burden, or the impact of the illness on the family or society.

Adjusting for severity is an essential step in performance improvement studies. Two patients with the same diagnosis may still present significant historical and clinical differences. If data used for comparative studies are not adjusted for the severity of the patients' illnesses, misleading or inaccurate comparisons may occur. The more heterogeneous the population studied, the greater the need to adjust for severity. Current methods of severity adjustment do not account for all differences between patients. A key challenge for the clinical knowledge worker is to understand and confront the limitations of various severity adjustment models while continuing to search for better ones.

Systems to measure severity may be based on electronic data taken from codes on medical records. However, these codes were never intended for this purpose. The codes may not fully capture enough clinical factors to provide the precision necessary to measure the severity of a patient's illness. They do not reflect the timing of events. And they fail to adjust risk based on admission severity. All these issues add to the inherent weakness of coded data for measuring care. Other systems employ clinical data manually abstracted from the medical record. The abstraction process is both costly and subject to human error and subjective interpretations.

In spite of the limitations of coding, stratifying patient groups by diagnosis or procedure can create more homogeneous groups. Patients who have identical procedures or diagnostic codes will be more similar to one another than patients in a diagnosis related group (DRG). But even at the ICD-9 level, adjustment must be made for comorbidities or additional diagnoses. In cases where a highly homogeneous patient group is under study, the need to adjust may be reduced. An example would be a study of all normal vaginal deliveries, with an operational definition that excludes all patients with risk factors.

What are the implications of failure to adjust data for severity? Serious problems may fail to be identified, and less serious problems then become the focus of investigation. Variation may be observed where it does not exist and may not be observed where it does exist. Physicians may lose confidence in profiling data. Time and energy spent on providing robust and clinically derived methods of severity adjustment lead to more accurate targeting of opportunities for improvement.

The Limitations of Administrative Data

In the search for severity adjustment, the clinical knowledge worker has two tasks: to find data and to find a way to adjust for severity, understanding the limitations of the methodology used. The most important limiting issue in adjusting data for severity is the source of the data.

The cost of acquiring clinical information for quality assessment has stimulated the use of less expensive administrative data sets (Iezzoni, 1997). The Office of Technology Assessment has stated that administrative data sets are limited in their ability to evaluate the comparative effectiveness of medical treatment (Office of Technology Assessment, 1994).

Administrative data come from federal and state governmental agencies, claims, and provider-sponsored organizations. The advantages of administrative data are that they are readily available, relatively inexpensive, computer readable, and encompass large populations. Because of these advantages, they are increasingly used for physician profiling and examination of practice variations. However, administrative data have significant limitations when used to measure quality. Gaps in clinical information in administrative data, due to coding nuances, inaccuracies, or incomplete information, may produce misleading results when measuring clinical care processes and outcomes. Problems with denominator reliability may result in inaccuracy of measurement, especially when using rate-based performance indicators. Administrative data do not fully address processes of care, errors, timing, appropriateness, or severity.

Although a more clinically robust source of data is needed for performance measurement, organizations typically make a trade-off between desirability and feasibility in their quest for relevant data. Iezzoni (1997) has noted that quality evaluation must be multidimensional whereas administrative data are capable of measuring only some dimensions and units of quality. She predicts that the scope and definitions for administrative data sets will change dramatically over the next several years. This prediction, in fact, appears to be accurate, as organizations and clinicians are suggesting richer, more robust measures of quality and at the same time searching for cost effectiveness and for the best methods to adjust for severity the administrative data sets currently available to them.

The first imperative for those involved in the measurement of care and performance improvement is to understand the limitations of administrative data and use them accordingly. Those preparing data for public consumption have a responsibility to describe their limitations.

Evaluating a Severity Adjustment System

An organization should approach the decision to purchase a severity of illness information system systematically, justifying the expenses and resources needed. To effectively select a severity-adjusting system, consideration must be given to validity and discriminating power.

Because data for performance initiatives involve multiple functions, personnel levels, and departments, a broad constituency of users should be engaged to identify the requirements of the system and the business processes it will support. Using a team approach in this effort builds consensus.

First, the individuals and constituencies that will own, implement, use, or have interest in the system should be identified and enlisted. The team should then define the requirements and create the business model for using the data results. In the search for the best system, the entire team should evaluate technical, economic, operational, and schedule feasibility and the strength of the potential vendor candidates.

A preimplementation audit can identify priorities and outline the requirements and intended benefits of the system. When conducted by the team, the audit can identify previously unforeseen issues and help the entire group rethink original assumptions about use of the data. The team selects the best system for the organization using the following steps.

Goals and Objectives

First, the team should articulate the business objectives of the system. Examples of these internal objectives are physician profiling, clinical practice improvement, resource utilization analysis, and benchmarking. Specific needs in outcomes management and resource management should be described as completely as possible. For example, one health care system developed the following succinct and clear goal for its system: "The system we select must assign a score to each patient record and provide our health care system the ability to insert this score directly into our data repository."

Operational Scope

An accurate and shared vision of the project scope is critical for implementation. One element to be defined here is the number of entities the system will need to serve. For example, will it include data for both inpatients and outpatients? The number of discharges or patient encounters the system will need to process is a key metric. A common pitfall in selecting a system is the failure to fully define the scope of the project or the failure to communicate a change in scope.

Organizational Readiness

An organization must be ready to install, support, and use the system. This may require changes in business practices. The impact of the system will extend beyond the quality and information management departments to virtually every department that processes clinical transactions. The adequacy of source systems and the data contained in them must be evaluated.

In addition, the installation of a severity of illness system requires reevaluation of the organization's coding requirements. Comorbidities and other conditions that affect risks must be coded. Because medical record codes rely on clinicians' written documentation, documentation practice may need to be supported. The implementation of a severity of illness system is often a catalyst for an organization's move to a structured medical record system and common vocabulary. Organizations frequently underestimate the interorganizational impact of severity of illness system implementation. A preimplementation audit of source systems and coding identifies at the onset of the project potential data validity and business process challenges.

Functional Requirements

A severity of illness system should have flexible, user-defined parameters. The calculation method of the severity algorithm and such key factors as the number of codes used for adjustment should be determined. Assessment of patient function includes assigning risk weights to various physiological factors, based on diagnosis. For example, does high blood pressure have one weight for pneumonia and a different weight for congestive heart failure? The statistical validity, reliability, and accuracy of these adjustments is important. If the system relies on discharge coding, how does it differentiate between discharge conditions and conditions evident on admission? If the system adjusts for multiple comorbidities, what factors determine the weighting?

The team should examine the ability of the severity system to track outcomes by episode or encounter on a longitudinal basis. The issue of database security must be addressed, and the ability of the system to limit access based on need to know should be ascertained. Most severity of illness systems can easily export data into statistical analysis packages. The variable inputs or interfaces required to perform this should be identified.

Ongoing Staff Requirements

The availability of training and support is a critical success factor in implementing a severity of illness system. Ongoing support requirements must be evaluated.

Technical Requirements

The processes for extracting hospital data, loading or submitting data into the system, defining aggregates and accumulations, and creating reports should be determined. The technical specifications of the system—hardware, software, operating system, database engine, programming languages, and optional configurations— should also be identified.

Timeline

The team should determine the date the system must be in place. Based on that date, it should set key milestone dates to achieve the goal. Team consensus and buy-in increase the likelihood that deadlines will be met. It is necessary to assess both the organization's and the vendor's ability to meet these deadlines.

Project Budget

The team should calculate one-time expenses, ongoing costs, and return on investment.

Potential Vendors

The team should begin seeking vendors by preparing a request for information (RFI) or request for proposal (RFP). This document communicates the features desired in a system and asks potential suppliers to provide a financial profile, installation history, list of clients by size, and information about the vendor company mission, vision, and plan for the future. A vendor's response should include a method to address each of the organization's key requirements.

Structured Vocabulary

Standardized vocabulary is important to the development of clinically detailed severity systems. A structured vocabulary is a selected set of specialized terms that facilitate precise communication. Controlled vocabularies are unambiguous, sharable, and can be aggregated.

The lack of standards for health care and clinical logic is a major obstacle in the development of clinically relevant decision support systems. This is also true of the development of severity systems. Standards for health care data are under way and are likely to emerge in the area of structured vocabularies (Broverman, 1999). Efforts to apply the reference clinical information model to clinical decision support are being made through HL7, which is an American National Standards Institute accredited body dedicated to information exchange among health care systems.

Clinicians will be well served by conforming to vocabulary standardization efforts, because this vocabulary will better document their effectiveness and marketability. However, these efforts are works in progress. Until a structured vocabulary is widely available, it is important for teams to answer three questions when finding and using administrative data to measure processes, outcomes, and effectiveness of care:

- Are the data adjusted?
- If so how? What methods are used?
- What are the implications of these methods for clinical knowledge workers who use the data?

Conclusion

Adjustment of health care data for severity is an important and often expensive consideration for health care organizations. Although administrative data today remain the most economical and more widely available source of data for performance improvement, they have limitations for discerning differences in patients' measurement of clinical quality. As a result, clinical workers search for more clinically rich sources of data to fully reflect clinical characteristics of patients in order to more accurately measure quality of care. Clinical knowledge workers must understand the limitations of administrative data and available systems of severity adjustment in order to use data appropriately.

The selection and purchase of an information system to severity adjust health care data is effectively accomplished by a team approach that addresses issues such as objectives of the system, operational scope, organizational readiness, technical requirements, extraction processes, implementation timelines, budget constraints, and systematic evaluation of potential vendors. Severity adjustment of health care data is enabled by standardization of vocabulary that uses a consistent set of terms to facilitate precise communication.

Chapter Nine

Integrating Clinical Information for Performance Improvement

In an integrated health care delivery system,
information technology is more than a tool.
Information flow is an essential part of the care
delivery process itself. This chapter explains why
clinical integration must include information and
how this information improves care.

We saw in Chapter One that clinical integration is the degree to which clinical services are coordinated across levels of care over time to achieve optimal cost and quality outcomes. Clinical integration is a key characteristic of high-performing organized delivery systems (Shortell, Gillies, Anderson, Mitchell, & Morgan, 1993). However, before care can be integrated, information must be integrated. To understand this, we need to examine the role of information in an integrated health care delivery system.

The relationship between information technology and clinical integration is synergistic and interdependent. The creation of clinically integrated information environments simultaneously supports and creates clinically integrated care processes. The key elements of clinical integration that accelerate process improvement are alignment of information system goals with the business goals of the organization, integration of quality models and processes across the continuum of care, and development of a clinical data model. In the clinically integrated health care system the site of care becomes less relevant as the flow of information between patient and clinician becomes smooth, efficient, and processed in real time.

Information Exchange in the Collaborative Community

Clinical integration and performance improvement both require intense and dynamic communication, team building, and innovation. The clinical knowledge community should encourage and expect learning, risk-taking, and discovery. Information must flow freely. As information increases, knowledge grows, and improvements are born.

As clinicians become more pressured by time, their need for information becomes more urgent. Internal and external networks depend on information. As information improves, clinical knowledge workers are able to access that better information to deliver care. Improvements in the capture and flow of information occur simultaneously with improvements in the process of care delivery. In this sense, information management is care management.

A key characteristic of the clinical knowledge community is the reduction of non-value-added activity. The creation of a consistent data model and common data definitions reduces non-value-added data capture and expensive, redundant data stores. Clinically integrated data models streamline the data collection process and ultimately the care delivery process. Clinical knowledge workers are thus free to focus on data necessary to improve care.

Key data for a patient include demographic information, past history and treatment, results of diagnostic testing, treatment plans, and information about encounters throughout the health care system. The integrated patient record ideally combines these elements into a unified whole, which is easily accessible to clinicians. Currently, these data are contained in a variety of disparate sources. Gathering them is part of the care process. The clinical interview is recognized as an integral part of the care process. The automation of data collection is simply an extension of the patient interview, employing technology and decision rules. Various forms of alerts and reminders delivered to caregivers become important components of building quality in at the front end of information system integration and deployment.

Goals and Approaches of Integrated Systems

The goal of a clinically integrated information system is to support the clinical knowledge community by enabling the transformation of data into information, which becomes knowledge to deliver and improve care. As the organization moves to a population-based, cross-continuum approach, information system planning must expand its scope and address the measurement of care as it occurs in complex and longitudinal episodes, not as though it were a series of loosely connected encounters.

The approach to clinical integration of data systems begins with a definition of the scope of clinical integration, identification of baseline status, and consideration of a number of possible business scenarios that information systems may need to support. A cluster of business, clinical, and storage applications comprise the core and will best equip integrated delivery systems regardless of business priorities. These applications are

- A clinical repository or data warehouse
- A master patient index or unique patient identifier that functions across all enterprise entities
- Scheduling, patient accounting, order entry, and clinical applications (such as pharmacy, laboratory, and clinical documentation applications) and applications that support nursing and care path and case management

Quality Management and Information Management

Quality improvement and information integration support and accelerate each other in the integrated health care network. Business functions such as quality management, utilization management, care coordination, outcomes management, call centers, regulatory compliance, and medical staff credentialing can all be improved by the process of information technology redesign. Data derived from these business functions must be combined to present a picture of the care of patients across the continuum.

Clinical integration initiatives focus on episodes and populations instead of encounters. Quality improvement must use information technology as a key tool when studying these integrated processes and outcomes of care. In order to collect integrated data sets, it may be necessary to structurally reorganize the traditional network of quality assurance and quality improvement initiatives by developing systemwide quality management oversight groups, cross-continuum models of care management, common credentialing, protocols and outcomes management, and the development of a comprehensive method of easy access for both patients and providers.

Several key methods are used to redesign quality management in a clinical integrated system. The first is development of an automated medical record across the health care enterprise and the development of valid and reliable clinical data. These integrated data are supported by information systems that make the data accessible to clinical knowledge workers. A key feature of quality redesign is an electronic linkage connecting patients and providers across the continuum of care. Additional defining features are clinical decision support systems, the deployment of practice profiling information to providers, and emergence of data-driven disease management.

The process of development of a pathway of care illustrates that as the need to cross the continuum increases, efforts to integrate data sources and collection also intensify. Efforts are directed at coordinating encounters of care, linking levels of acute and subacute care, coordinating care across the life span, and coordinating specialty services within a system (Conrad, 1993). These efforts are directed at integration of clinical data but have the additional benefit of accelerating quality improvement efforts. Measurement of the care of broad bases of populations is necessary in order to evaluate true outcomes and to know what makes care better. Both information gathering activities and knowledge-based activities are part of the quality improvement process.

Information technology must be clinically integrated to communicate with all levels of care that a patient may need to move through, such as social services, rehabilitation, acute care, visiting nurse or home care, and primary and specialist care follow-up. Referrals and outcomes of care must be documented at each step; detailed reports ideally must be available to providers before the patient arrives. The patient and family should have the expectation that the health care system already knows about their needs. Continuum care management requires data support across clinical pathways. The clinically integrated information system incorporates outcome data collection with the utilization management and care management process and interfaces to a computerized medical record and to patient clinical pathways.

Information systems supporting care improvement should provide reporting on path variance, discharge planning, case manager workload, productivity, and resource consumption and should be designed to allow monitoring of these variables. Other data elements important in the care management process include home conditions, patient and family concerns, patient ability to handle daily living tasks, and patient and family preferences and special needs. The ideal clinically integrated system should allow all participants in patient care management to access information based on their need to know and should provide appropriate security and access control. The clinically integrated information system is multiuser and multientity. Data integrity provisions should start at input screens, and strict data validity standards and business procedures and edits that support these standards should be established. The development of the information environment to support this activity requires changes in business processes and organizational structure.

Conclusion

As integrated delivery systems search for and use integrated clinical data, care is not just measured but improved. The process of real-time data capture of the clinical elements necessary for integrated data systems necessitates changes in care delivery processes, from uncoordinated, subjective, and intuitive to coordinated, quantitative, and evidence based. This new process becomes the idealized, clinically integrated design. The flow of information becomes both an enabler of care improvement and part of the care process itself. As the clinical knowledge worker identifies the important data elements to capture in evaluating the process of care, care is increasingly monitored, and key quality goals are defined. The case study that follows in Chapter Ten illustrates the strategy and challenges of system deployment in an integrated health care enterprise.

Chapter Ten

Case Study

Linking and Integrating Enterprisewide Health Information Management Data

Donna Bowers

Health information management can seem like a
formidable task, particularly in large organizations
with multiple sites. This case study shows how one
health care system automated and standardized
tasks and made important improvements in
transcription, chart management, and clinical
abstracting. The chapter also examines how
these integrated systems are paving the way for
enterprisewide access to information via the
intranet or Internet. These improvements have
made it easier for clinical knowledge workers to
access data.

Keeping pace with the changes in health care is difficult, costly, and
challenging. Transforming the health information management
(HIM) department is a lot like trying to build a better boat when
you are already far out to sea. To avoid sinking, you can't tear your
ship apart before you have something else to replace it. You must

keep the ship afloat by managing today's priorities while constructing the new ship by selecting and implementing new systems. New technology and solutions surely bring the computerized patient record within sight, yet there are many obstacles to overcome before we can get there safely, such as maintaining productivity and service while bringing in the new system, training staff, managing costs, and aligning efforts with corporate strategies and enterprise business goals. A carefully thought out strategy is needed.

Most facilities today face the challenge of migrating patient data in paper form to electronic data. At Baylor Health Care System (BHCS), the issues along the way are challenging and complex. The purpose of this chapter is to review some of the strategies and methods used successfully at Baylor University Medical Center (BUMC) to link and integrate patient data across the enterprise, particularly in the HIM department.

The Perfect Information Solution

In a perfect world an enterprisewide health care information management system would have common applications from a single vendor, all feeding data to a single data repository. Unified data fields and definitions would be the standard rather than the exception. Access to information would be based on a business or clinical need, and the health care information system would require minimal upkeep. Data would be shared across the continuum of care as a matter of practice for delivering high-quality care to the patient. The perfect information solution would also mean that implementation of such a system could be implemented today— now—not at some point in the future.

The Imperfect Information Reality

The reality at Baylor—and at many health care organizations across the country—is that a perfect enterprisewide solution does not yet exist for an organization with multiple facilities and multiple points of access. Although some information is shared between facilities, in many cases the data flow in one direction only, and there are some facilities with no connection at all to other facilities.

To meet today's pressing needs, health care organizations are using systems from a variety of developers and pushing interface technology to the fullest. To make matters more complicated, HIM professionals have to contend with migrating older systems to newer technologies, cope with current workload and processing needs, and carefully plan for the future—all at the same time. There are more projects on the table than there are qualified HIM and information systems staff to bring them to fruition.

A Key to Implementing the Electronic Medical Record

One of the keys to the successful implementation of the electronic medical record is to ensure that the best possible automation is in place and functioning successfully. Many factors play a role in making decisions critical to the success of the enterprise. The hardware and the software must work in concert and meet the current needs as well as be strategically placed for the future. The right hardware needs the right software and vice versa: one without the other can result in delays or, in some cases, failures.

The systems chosen and the processes engineered will have a direct impact on patient care and the continued competitiveness and viability of the enterprise. HIM and information systems have to work closely together. With competition as tight as it is and the dwindling of financial resources, costly mistakes are not easily absorbed or overlooked.

The health care market is no longer what it once was. Market pressures are forcing health care providers such as the Baylor enterprise to expand, to provide more comprehensive services, and to include more and more of the community's health care professionals in response to the cost-cutting pressures placed on hospitals by payers—health maintenance organizations, preferred provider organizations, and such. As providers expand they must find ways of taking advantage of that expansion by leveraging resources as much as possible.

The critical point is that the HIM department must continue to maintain a high level of service and support to physicians, to other health care providers, and especially to patients. Short-term and long-term strategies must coexist so that the level of service expected by the providers in the enterprise will not be compromised. At the same time, the bridges to the next levels of automation must be built so that the transition will be smooth and successful.

Overview of the Baylor Health Care System

The Baylor Health Care System is one of the largest health care networks in the nation, providing a comprehensive range of services to the population of Dallas and its surrounding areas and to patients throughout Texas and the Southwest region.

The Baylor network consists of several medical centers, over twelve senior health centers, one rehabilitation facility, three subacute adult and pediatric centers, home health services, private physician practices, and major medical research facilities. More than sixteen hundred physicians are affiliated with Baylor.

The flagship of Baylor Health Care System is BUMC, a full-service tertiary teaching hospital. Located on a thirty-two-block campus in downtown Dallas, it comprises five connecting hospitals.

Network Infrastructure

Eight hospitals and numerous health care delivery sites are connected directly to the network and share data across the enterprise network. Within each facility, a fiber optics network is being installed to replace the existing network infrastructure. Baylor is currently engaged in connecting the remaining sites to the central network via LAN and WAN technology. Redundant T-1 lines are being used to connect all remote facilities.

Now and in the foreseeable future the core HIM applications and systems will operate on standard PC hardware connected via the Novell network operating system. Today there is a mix of DOS and Windows applications, and a process of converting DOS-based applications to Windows is under way as they become available and practical.

Many of the evolutionary changes in HIM start at the BUMC facility, the largest center in BHCS. Once a new system has proven successful there, the strategy is to implement it across the enterprise where practical—according to budget, staffing, and implementation resource schedules.

Transcription

The transcribed report is the most important piece of clinical information in the patient record. Transcribed reports are the foundation for the data repository, making up the majority of the content of the patient record. The key indicators of success for transcription are quality and accuracy of documentation, turnaround time, and especially, access to physician reports.

Previously, transcription at BHCS was performed on disparate systems with no interconnectivity between facilities. Today, the entire enterprise is moving toward a common transcription vendor. At the downtown Baylor facilities, all transcription for all inpatient and outpatient reports except radiology and pathology is done on the same system. Transcribed reports are available on-line seven days a week. Completed reports are transferred to a centralized optical disk server, where they remain available permanently.

Staffing management is made much easier through the centralized system. Transcriptionists use the same system to create almost every report so that training is much quicker. Close to one hundred separate report types are created through the transcription system.

The Microsoft Word–based transcription system at BUMC is integrated with the dictation system through a digital dictation system interface, which provides the transcriptionists with data about the dictating physician, the patient, and the document type. The transcription system shares an interface with the Eclipsys host system at BUMC, which provides further patient demographic and admission data to transcriptionists. These data elements are entered into the report where appropriate. We have a first-time 85 percent match rate between the medical record number keyed in by the dictating physician and the information held on the host system. Considering the volume of documents created every day, we consider this a highly successful system.

BUMC transcriptionists handle the work for all the downtown Dallas facilities, including the Baylor Center for Restorative Care, Our Children's Home, and the senior health centers. Transcription is done seven days a week with at least two shifts a day. Production levels are at sixty thousand dictation minutes per month.

Further integration allows the chart deficiency analysis system to automatically note the dictation job and the transcription job. The electronic signature application product used by physicians also automatically updates the chart completion matrix.

Document Distribution

Getting the report back to the physicians contributes significantly to their ability to provide quality patient care. Physicians receive their reports and copies through a third-party distribution system that integrates with the transcription system. Most physicians receive reports on their office PCs.

Additionally, the transcription system includes an add-on module for managing batch printing of reports to appropriate network printers at the various locations throughout the system. The system prints reports at prescheduled times.

Original reports are printed in the HIM department for placement in the patient's chart upon discharge.

Document Storage

All transcribed reports are archived on-line through an optical platter storage system. The archive system allows the documents to be available without having to retrieve patients' medical records.

Electronic Document Signature

BUMC has implemented an electronic signature system that is integrated with the transcription system and the chart deficiency management system. The Windows-based PC system allows physicians to review, edit, and sign their dictated reports. It is available from any of the strategically placed workstations in the dining room, operating room area, and physician signing area of the HIM department. Physicians also have access to their documents from their offices.

The integrated system provides on-line access to dictated reports. In addition, the chart deficiency management system is automatically updated with each signed report. In many cases a report can be logged by the deficiency management module—from dictation and transcription to signature—without intervention by the HIM staff, and the physician gets full credit for the work. All of the physicians felt that patient care was positively affected because of improved document integrity.

In a recent survey of physicians using the system, 100 percent of the respondents were happy with the system and would recommend it to a colleague; 80 percent said the electronic signature system reduced the number of visits needed to the HIM department. At BUMC we are encouraged by the physicians' response to the automation and by their willingness to be directly involved in the documentation process.

Electronic Signature via the Internet

Emerging Internet and intranet technologies present tremendous opportunities for HIM departments to provide even greater levels of accurate, timely, and cost-efficient service to their enterprises.

Internet and intranet technology offers the potential to revolution-
ize the HIM field, and it is most likely that health care organizations
will probably have no choice but to embrace this technology to
remain competitive in the future.

BUMC is currently undergoing final testing to provide access
to the electronic signature system via the Internet or Baylor's
intranet. With this application, physicians will have the ability to
review, edit, and sign documents on-line from virtually anywhere,
with the distinct advantage of not having to learn a new system.
The Internet version of the electronic signature program will have
the same look and feel and functionality as its network counterpart.
Additionally, any software updates to the electronic signature system will be managed by the server at BUMC and pushed along to
the physician user when he or she logs on.

The key enabling technology for this application is a Weblink
server dedicated to the task of managing electronic signature sessions over the Internet or BUMC's intranet. The Weblink server
handles database transactions and back-end processing to help
minimize the data throughput along the network.

To access the application via the Internet, the physician must
first connect to the Internet by using an Internet service provider.
Once a dial-up connection has been established, the physician
launches the electronic signature application, which automatically
establishes a connection to BUMC's Internet server and then to
the electronic signature Weblink server. The physician must enter
a valid user name and password once to connect to the Internet
server and then once again for access to the electronic signature
application. Only the physician knows his or her own password.
Naturally, document security is a major issue here, and we feel this
solution provides reasonable security measures.

Chart Management

With the frequent need for patient charts to travel within the
enterprise, a centralized chart management system is used at four of
the Dallas facilities—BUMC, Baylor Center for Restorative Care,

Baylor Institute for Rehabilitation, and Our Children's Home. The system allows HIM staff to check charts in and out of these facilities so that HIM staff know where a chart is at all times.

An integrated release of information module allows BUMC to control the release of information process even though we contract the work to an outside vendor. The same database is used at the four downtown facilities.

Clinical Abstracting, Quality Assurance, and Utilization Management

For historical reasons, such as different facilities using different medical record schemes and different mainframe host systems, BHCS does not use an enterprise master person index, which further complicates efforts to integrate data between facilities. However, by using the most up-to-date technology to develop a common database, Baylor has been able to link the data between facilities without using an enterprise master person index. Clinical abstracts from three Baylor facilities are stored in the central archive database, which is housed at the main Baylor facility. An archive system is used to interact with clinical abstracting to allow for document storage and immediate on-line availability. A fourth facility, Baylor Medical Center at Irving, is currently working on the implementation plan for connecting to the database.

In July 1996, the new clinical abstract system was implemented at three Baylor facilities: BUMC, Baylor Center for Restorative Care, and Our Children's Home. Along with clinical abstracting, the system includes integrated modules for quality assurance (QA) and utilization management (UM), both of which were previously managed via a paper-based system.

An important component of this configuration is a PC-based on-line archive system, which allows archived data from the data collection modules—clinical abstract, QA, and UM—to be archived in the same location. Abstract records are primarily financially driven, based on patient encounters, with QA and UM records for each patient tied to the patient encounter. Clinical abstract, QA, and UM patient records share core patient demographic data elements as well as data such as admitting diagnosis, working DRG, procedure codes, and subsequent diagnosis codes, with cross-references to the physicians and other patient caregivers. This greatly increases system accuracy and efficiency, yet each module contains specific data elements and input screens designed for the function at hand. Further, the system provides security options so that clinical abstract, QA, and UM staff have access to only the system areas that they need; this prevents unauthorized access to sensitive information. The real advantage to having an on-line archive is that the number of records in the active clinical abstract, QA, and UM databases is kept to a minimum. At Baylor, abstract records are moved to the archive product after sixty days so that the active system is at peak performance levels at all times.

Baylor had twelve years of historical clinical abstract data in its repository. On implementation, data for the last five years were loaded into the new archive product. The remaining seven years of data were loaded to an off-line repository. Currently, more than forty thousand records are added each month, and the archive holds close to one million patient episode records. Along with the new abstracting system, the three facilities began coding both inpatient and outpatient episodes. In the first year alone, there was a 258 percent increase in the number of patient records created.

Installation of the new abstracting system gave Baylor the chance to redesign its abstract database from scratch. Over time, some data fields had become redundant yet were still being captured. A special committee was formed with representatives from the three original facilities, including UM and QA representatives, to establish a common data dictionary. Each field, each screen, and each report was carefully examined to determine whether it was still needed. Eventually, the team was able to agree on each field, each item, and each table.

Because Baylor's experience with the integrated data collection system has been so successful, the plan is to replace any abstracting system at Baylor facilities with the one being used at BUMC, Baylor Center for Restorative Care, and Our Children's Home. The committee process continues today, with Baylor Medical Center at Irving, the second largest facility in BHCS, scheduled to come online with the system, bringing the total number of facilities to six. The same committee serves as a triage for requests for new data elements so that new fields can be implemented uniformly, taking Baylor's "big-picture" needs into account. Only through careful and consistent maintenance of the database can it continue to support the evolving needs of the enterprise.

The key to tying the data together enterprisewide was the introduction of a "site ID" field in the data record. The site ID field allows us to produce reports on an individual facility or aggregate facility basis.

Integrating Utilization Management and Quality Assurance

With the introduction of the new clinical abstracting system, Baylor's UM and QA departments gained a new level of automation and efficiencies through the integrated modules.

Using an interface engine, we are able to bring real-time patient demographic data to coders and to UM and QA case reviewers. Not only does this save tremendous data entry time, with data being entered only once at the source and used many times throughout the facility, but the improvement in accuracy is dramatic. Using laptop computers, case reviewers have real-time access to data on the unit floors where they perform their work.

The modules support the use of clinical pathway management termed *care paths* at Baylor. The integrated system provides a wealth of reports, many of which were not possible previously. Case mix reports, QA and UM reports, trends and variances, avoidable days and reasons, and also physician credentials are available from the same applications. The systems also complement tumor and trauma registries, serving as the main feed of data to those areas for case finding, management, and follow-up.

The integrated abstracting, QA, and UM system has proven to be even more reliable than similar reports we were getting from the host system; so those ADT (admissions, discharge, transfer) reports have been eliminated now that the clinical abstracting system has more current data.

Through the use of a batch printing scheduling program, many of the reports that need to be generated daily or weekly are done so automatically. QA and UM review logs, for example, are printed automatically and made available to case reviewers at the nursing stations each morning.

On-Line Medical Record Viewing

In addition to electronic signature, BUMC is in the process of delivering a medical record viewing application for physicians, which will provide on-line viewing access to patient documentation from workstations on the LAN, WAN, Internet, and intranet. It is an interim solution to a host-system-based electronic medical record, with the primary goal of eliminating as much paper as possible, particularly in outpatient and emergency department service areas.

The viewing tool integrates data and documents from core systems such as the transcription system and also from the radiology and laboratory systems.

The Internet version of this system will employ the same dedicated Weblink technology as the electronic signature application. Again, the look and feel and functionality will be identical to that of other means of access for the physician users of the system.

Conclusion

The HIM department at BUMC and throughout BHS is leading the way in automation and integration in this field. For many years the HIM department was viewed as a holding place for paper. In today's environment, however, HIM is working toward a computerized medical record for the future while developing ways to auto-mate and provide access to it.

The strategies discussed in this chapter are all supporting Bay-lor's direction and planning. It is critical that systems are selected that can perform at desired levels today and can integrate and grow with future designs. At Baylor the word *partnership* is not a cliché. Only through true partnerships between departments, vendors, and systems will we be able to keep our ship sailing smoothly into the future.

Chapter Eleven

Case Study

Drilling Down for
Performance Improvement Data

Annette Rowton
Susan McBride

Clinical knowledge workers use many techniques
to extract integrated clinical and financial data
from the databases available to them. This chapter
uses a case study to discuss how clinical knowledge
workers integrate data from a variety of source
systems and use business application software to
promote immediate interaction with clinicians and
analysts in order to increase data support for their
fast-track continuous quality improvement efforts.

The analysis of patterns of care requires extraction of data elements from a variety of clinical, financial, and other data sources. One of the greatest challenges for today's clinical knowledge workers is obtaining line item detail about the cost and quality of care. Cost accounting or billing data reside in financial databases. Rich clinical information resides in records manually abstracted by clinical knowledge workers or in department-based clinical databases. The manual process required to combine and then aggregate these data is time and resource intensive.

Clinical knowledge workers use many techniques to facilitate and expedite the query process. Here are the steps in a typical study query process:

1. Determine the study question or hypothesis.
2. Precisely define the study population, using a specific clinical characteristic or a diagnosis related group (DRG), ICD-9, or CPT code.
3. Secure necessary approvals for release of and access to the data.
4. Identify the data period to be studied.
5. Identify the source systems for the data.
6. Identify potential limitations of the database sources.
7. Identify severity adjustment mechanisms and their limitations.
8. Prepare the output report format.
9. Harvest the data from the various source systems using identical populations and qualifiers.
10. Check the denominator of patients from each system. Reconcile any differences in patient counts in each system before proceeding.
11. Integrate the data from the source systems. This step often requires mapping the different data sources to one another. There must be a common data element or unique identifier(s) that allows one-to-one mapping of the different data sources so that a particular episode of care is identified accurately. Examples of patient characteristics that are often used are encounter numbers, medical record number combined with date of admission, or date of procedure.
12. Download the data into a spreadsheet or database application for manipulation or sorting.
13. Compute statistical analysis, such as measures of central tendency, with standard deviations and severity scores.

14. Maintain all files for final audit.
15. Prepare a report in the report template.
16. Audit the report for accuracy as each of the above steps is completed.
17. Revise the report as needed.
18. Label for confidentiality as appropriate.

The steps in this process are cumbersome for an analyst who needs data rapidly to measure the effectiveness of a performance improvement initiative. Methods to streamline the query process can be developed by clinical knowledge workers until an information environment to support real-time performance improvement is implemented.

The Data Challenge in a Large Health Care System

The quality managers in a large health care system needed increased data analysis capability to support fast-track clinical process improvement. Traditional process improvement efforts typically take four to six months, whereas fast-track efforts aim for results in six to eight weeks. The rate limiting steps are often the data analysis and reporting requirements. Additionally, sufficient clinical detail is often lacking in readily available data sources. This example addresses both of these challenges.

This particular health care system uses data from the cost accounting system to identify opportunities for improvement in resource utilization. The health care system's cost accounting application groups items at the product level. This level of data often lacks sufficient clinical detail. Although many studies effectively identify variations in practice patterns (resource utilization) with this level of detail, other studies are hampered by the inability to drill down into more specifics.

For example, in a study of laparoscopic cholecystectomy, it was necessary to obtain sufficient data detail to analyze key resource utilization drivers and to analyze potential variation among providers. After exhausting the cost accounting system as a source of information, other systems were queried for additional detail, including the admissions, discharge, and transfer (ADT) system; surgical databases; and other clinical databases. This process, illustrated in Figure 11.1, required labor-intensive mapping of ICD-9 codes and integration of data. In one system these information and data elements were coded as numbers. In another they were coded as letters. In both cases, the variable was first translated into one type (letters or numbers) before conversion could take place. Although these data drills were all eventually successful, they were time consuming and frustrating for the clinical knowledge workers, who wanted to spend value-added time analyzing the data.

The Information Processing Environment

The health care system is composed of five system-owned hospitals, three affiliated hospitals, and over twenty-five outpatient centers, including rural, senior, and emergent care centers. The information system environment consists of a single wide-area network, which delivers 230 applications to more than 2,300 networked devices; personal computers operate as universal workstations. The network connects thirty-five locations over a 120-mile diameter.

In 1991, the information services division decided to pursue an open systems approach, far more difficult and complex than its mainframe tradition. The commitment to open systems conferred upon the users the opportunity to select best-of-market applications to serve their needs.

The difficulty of open systems is integration. To facilitate communication between disparate systems, a complex, sophisticated interface engine was installed. The interface engine allows data collected in one system to be shared with multiple systems without user intervention. The delivery of information services is dependent on the efforts of application experts in the user community. These superusers are experts in specific applications, and they provide the first line of support to end users.

Figure 11.1. Previous Data Analysis Methodology.

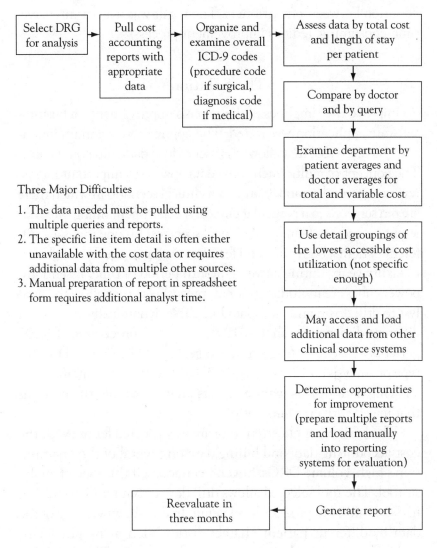

Select DRG for analysis → Pull cost accounting reports with appropriate data → Organize and examine overall ICD-9 codes (procedure code if surgical, diagnosis code if medical) → Assess data by total cost and length of stay per patient ↓ Compare by doctor and by query ↓ Examine department by patient averages and doctor averages for total and variable cost ↓ Use detail groupings of the lowest accessible cost utilization (not specific enough) ↓ May access and load additional data from other clinical source systems ↓ Determine opportunities for improvement (prepare multiple reports and load manually into reporting systems for evaluation) ↓ Reevaluate in three months ← Generate report

Three Major Difficulties

1. The data needed must be pulled using multiple queries and reports.
2. The specific line item detail is often either unavailable with the cost data or requires additional data from multiple other sources.
3. Manual preparation of report in spreadsheet form requires additional analyst time.

One of the systems most frequently used by clinical knowledge workers is the cost accounting database. The system originally did not always provide sufficient detail description at the line-item level to determine practitioner variation in utilization. In order to obtain this information, analysts manually combined cost accounting data with billing data to drill down to an acceptable level of detail. Often multiple spreadsheets were created to analyze the variation between practitioners. The result was a labor-intensive, time-consuming, tedious improvement process.

The Solution

To improve the timelines of the process improvements, a business software application was tested. The application is a multidimensional analysis tool that allows the user to load data into power cubes. The concept of multidimensional data analysis is important for system users to understand. Consider a clinical scenario in which there are ten surgeons in a particular clinical specialty performing three different procedures (similar in clinical specifics) on one thousand different patients, both male and female, varying in age from eighteen to eighty years, during a twelve-month period of time. Essentially, power cubes are multidimensional spreadsheets that allow the analyst to drill down and view data like these dynamically, in all their different dimensions: that is, 10 surgeons × 3 procedures × 1,000 patients × 2 sexes × 6 age groups (ages should be grouped for this type of analysis) × 12 months = 4,320,000 different combinations. Viewing data in this manner assists analysts to identify patterns that may be drivers of utilization.

The business application software was selected for use with the cost accounting data and billing data on several of the organization's high-volume DRGs. Several vendors sell this type of analysis tool. The tool selected allows drill down from DRG, to ICD-9, to department, to product-level detail. It also allows viewing of the data by different patient characteristics, such as by physician-specific patient population, gender, and age group. This capability supports interactive data analysis in the continuous quality improvement process.

The tool is taken into group meetings to present findings and drill down for further explanations of the variations noted. The time clinical professionals have for participation in process improvement is often limited, yet it is critical to get their input during the analytical phase. The traditional process resulted in a time-consuming feedback loop. Paper reports or overheads were presented to the teams for input and direction, and subsequently analysts returned to the outcomes department to create additional queries from source systems, to manually integrate the data, and to create multiple spreadsheets in preparation for the next meeting to present findings. The turnaround time was generally one to six weeks for reporting and analysis alone, depending on the complexity of the analysis and intensity of efforts. This is an example of the rate limiting steps noted above.

This tool can be used for immediate interaction with clinicians and analysts. The software and power cubes can be taken into meetings via laptop for interactive analysis with the clinical professionals involved in the process. One issue that should be noted with this application is that the analysts must have a keen understanding of it and prior knowledge of the data in it before the interaction. There is a learning curve with multidimensional analysis techniques. The analyst who has traditionally used two-dimensional spreadsheets may need to relearn analytical thought processes and data drill-down techniques.

Additional considerations are data preparation and the information system. Several steps must occur prior to loading data into the power cubes, and they are critical elements of the process. Failure to properly prepare the data can result in inaccuracy and misleading information. The steps necessary for data preparation are as follows (also see Figure 11.2):

1. Harvest the data from the source systems and maintain files for data validation.

2. Integrate data from the systems, with careful attention to merging the data. Map the data appropriately, and recode them if necessary.

3. Compute any additional information that you may be interested in, such as means, modes, medians, and risk scores. A spreadsheet application, statistical package, or relational

Figure 11.2. New Data Analysis Methodology.

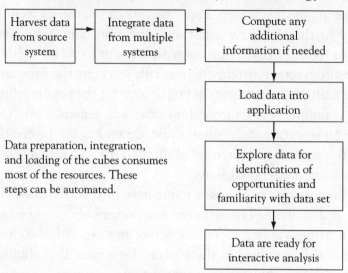

database may be used for this step. Maintain the files for validation.

4. Load the data into the transformer system and convert the data to power cubes. The analyst should consider power cube application limitations on size of files. Large data sets should be segmented into separate cubes for analysis. The separation should be based on clinical or operational determinations. An analysis might use one DRG per cube, for example, but this is highly variable, depending on the period of time to be examined and the number of admissions.

Multiple cubes can be connected for drill through from cube to cube. For example, if an analysis of percutaneous transluminal coronary angioplasty (PTCA) patients who require open-heart surgery was desired, the PTCA patients might be in one cube and the open-heart patients might be in another. The connection of cubes requires much more sophistication and is not recommended for the introduction of this analysis technique. The connection of cubes also requires substantial equipment. Data warehousing and client server environments are recommended when employing this capability, due to the size of the file structure required by multiple cubes.

Validity checks should be built into the process at each step to ensure accuracy of information.

The Results

Cardiac catheterizations, cardiac catheter laboratory interventions, total joint replacements, and lumbar and cervical discectomy cases were loaded into cubes for analysis and identification of improvement opportunities. Analysis revealed wide variation in the practice patterns of the lumbar discectomy and anterior cervical discectomy cases. This tool is excellent for identifying precisely what is driving the variation at an individual practitioner level, such as the high resource use associated with lumbar discectomy and anterior cervical discectomy cases using bone grafts and instrumentation.

Opportunities were identified for potential standardization of medication usage and of some products, such as PTCA balloons and stents, and joint prostheses. Day-of-the-week practice patterns were noted, with opportunities for improving scheduling routines in the operating room and cardiac catheter laboratory. Longer lengths of stay and time lags from date of admission to date of procedure were identified with patterns clustered around Friday, Saturday, and Sunday. The opportunity for better weekend use of the catheter laboratory and operating room could potentially decrease length of stay.

The analysis revealed information that could also have been derived by the previous methodology. The difference with the new methodology was that these discoveries took minutes to detect, rather than hours of paper report generation, fragmented analysis of multiple reports, and delay in delivering the results of the analysis.

Conclusion

To support real-time quality improvement work, today's quality analysts must streamline the steps used in this query-and-discovery process. These needs are especially acute in fast-track and accelerated improvement models.

Rich clinical and financial information resides in disparate databases in many health care organizations. The ideal clinically integrated information system is not yet a reality. Clinical knowledge workers must often use an iterative process of query and discovery to gather these data and then drill down to analyze patterns of care to understand clinical and cost outcomes.

Clinical knowledge workers in this case study illustrate a creative approach to a quest for integrated data as they employ a business application to support interactive data analysis and a fast-track quality improvement process. These workers demonstrate creative data quests that pioneer new ways to find and integrate data to support their quality improvement efforts.

Chapter Twelve

Case Study

Measuring the Effectiveness
of Clinical Pathways

Bonita Ann Pilon

Clinical knowledge workers often integrate data to
measure the effectiveness of clinical pathways, or
more specifically, the treatment regimen outlined
on the pathway. The clinical pathway assists
clinicians as a team to focus attention on key
variables. The case study in this chapter shows how
clinical knowledge workers use variance data to
complete a root cause analysis of variation. After
the analysis, appropriate action can be taken to
improve clinical outcomes.

The first question that must be answered is, What is the aim of the
pathway? Pathways are developed for many reasons, including
streamlining documentation, creating task lists for nurses, and
pleasing payers.

From a quality improvement perspective, clinical pathways are
designed and used for one important reason: to decrease variability by using the best available practice as identified by the clinical
management team. The process of pathway development—exploring current steps in the clinical management of targeted patients,
reviewing charts, researching the literature for best practices

(evidence-based medicine)—focuses the attention of clinicians on key process variables that were (perhaps) previously overlooked. For pneumonia patients, for example, the team may discover that there is great variability in the timing of the first antibiotic dose, which affects length of stay. When the pathway is written, the team will probably include measurement of an intermediate outcome, which captures whether the drug was initiated within the acceptable time frame.

Through the variance capture system, data are collected on key events that affect quality of care and resource utilization. Individual patient data are grouped into population data in order to inform the clinical management team how well the population met the treatment goals. The number of intermediate outcomes to be tracked should be limited to the most important process variables in the clinical management of the patient. One stroke management team discovered it was tracking four separate outcomes related to voiding independently over a seven-day length of stay. Nurses were asked to assess and record these data four times.

Capturing variance data related to outcomes is almost always the responsibility of the staff nurse. It is critical to guard against overburdening the nursing staff with documentation tasks. The clinical management team and quality department staff may need reminding from time to time that the purpose of the bedside nurse is not to collect data for a research study but to provide direct care to patients. Outcome measurement should be integrated into the clinical documentation system of the bedside care providers and not be redundant to it. Automated systems—clinical information systems—often allow effortless collection of variance and outcome data, but paper systems can also be designed that lighten the documentation burden on the nursing staff.

The key issues in deriving and using data from clinical pathways are data collection methods (that is, integrating the collection process into the clinical documentation system), careful selection of the key variables for tracking, a willing and able clinical management team to analyze data and make practice changes, and timely reporting of patterns and trends.

Data Variance in Clinical Pathways for CABG Patients

In a five-hundred-bed community tertiary medical center, the open-heart surgery program had used clinical pathways for all coronary artery bypass graft (CABG) and valve repair patients for more than five years. Intermediate goals were identified on the pathway for each day of stay, beginning with the first twelve hours postoperatively. These goals were linked to body systems, and the tasks that supported each goal were also listed on the pathway for the nurses and ancillary staff to follow as they cared for patients. When the goals were not achieved, the variance was documented in the clinical documentation system. Case managers analyzed aggregate variance data monthly and presented them to the clinical management team quarterly.

Over a two-month period, the case managers noticed that a number of goals related to hemodynamic stability and extubation were not being met on time. This was a change from previous months. In addition, the length of stay was increased on these same patients. This trend alone was sufficient to report to the clinical management team at the quarterly meeting. However, these data detectives also audited charts on the patients in order to decipher what had caused this unusual pattern. They discovered that approximately six patients each month had returned to the operating room for reentry procedures, thus affecting the intubation time, hemodynamic stability, and length of stay outcomes. The reason for reentry was excessive bleeding during the immediate postoperative period. The case managers, clinical experts in the care of these patients, knew that such an increase in reentries for bleeding was unusual for their patient population. They continued to look for patterns among the affected patients: Were these patients sicker (comorbidities) prior to surgery? Were these patients older than the average patient during the same time period? They discovered that these patients did not seem to have any preexisting condition that was predictive of problems.

As the data were drilled down, a common factor emerged among the affected patients: all received the same cardiac inotropic drug while in the operating room, which was continued in the intensive care unit. Again the data detectives needed more information: Did the other, unaffected patients receive the same drug? The same dosage? Did the drug have known side effects that included bleeding? Had the surgeons changed their practice recently to include the use of this drug during surgery?

They consulted the clinical pharmacist who confirmed that the drug could cause bleeding in some patients. They consulted with the surgeons and the operating room staff and learned that the drug had been introduced into routine usage in the past three months. The case managers then knew enough about the situation to present the data, based on variance from the pathway (recorded by the bedside staff nurses), to the clinical management team. They also invited the clinical pharmacist to attend the meeting in order to present data on the drug's side effects.

Data Sources

The data detectives analyzed data from several sources. The initial alert that patients were not meeting treatment goals came from the variance reporting system, an automated capture system that produced monthly reports to the case managers about how well the intermediate goals were achieved in the patient population. Chart audit was performed manually for the patients identified as having experienced unexpected outcomes. As the data were further developed, brief, informal interviews took place with the operating room staff and surgeons to determine if clinical practice had changed. Pharmacy charge data were derived from the financial system on a per case and aggregate basis. The integrators of these data were the case managers, who were able to synthesize diverse data elements as a result of their root cause analysis.

Discussion

This case study illustrates several important points about the use of clinical pathways. First, the effective monitoring of key processes and outcome variables imbedded in a clinical pathway can focus the clinical care team on opportunities for improvement very quickly. Second, systematic monitoring provides data upon which staff can make treatment decisions, rather than relying on speculation or opinion. Third, unexpected patterns require further drill down to fully reveal why the unexpected is happening. A control chart can pinpoint special cause variation (as seen in this case study), but root cause analysis is essential before improvements can be made. Fourth, it takes a team of experts to analyze all the data and make effective treatment decisions that will affect the entire population of patients. Data must be presented to the clinical team in an easily understandable format. That responsibility fell to the case managers in this case study example.

In their role as clinical experts and data detectives, the case managers pulled pathway-generated data together in a meaningful way, helping the larger team act on opportunities for improvement. In the beginning of their analysis, the case managers were data farmers, willing to work hard to drill down to get the information and, when necessary, willing to perform an adequate root cause analysis.

The pathway-generated data provided the case managers the initial alert that stimulated their data search. As they pursued their quest and drilled down for the root cause of the variation, they demonstrated the characteristic behavior of the data explorer as they relied heavily on iteration and ad hoc query. Finally, after improvements were made, monitoring had to continue to ensure that the change was, in fact, an improvement.

Conclusion

This case study is a very good example of the Plan, Do, Check, Act (PDCA) cycle applied to the behavior of clinical knowledge workers in performance improvement. The clinical pathway proved highly effective as an information tool in this case: it provided a consistent standard of care for this patient population, and the monitoring process for clinical outcomes predicted by the pathway alerted the team when action was needed to improve care. The integration of data by the case managers was a manual process and required extraction of data from a variety of sources as they both farmed for data and explored each query iteration.

Chapter Thirteen

Case Study

Integrating Clinical and Financial Data to Create a Balanced Scorecard

LaVone Neal
Jennifer Walker

Integrating clinical and financial data in a
balanced scorecard provides a visual snapshot of
the overall performance of a health care
organization. This case study illustrates how
developing a balanced scorecard requires
integration of data and how it can ultimately
enhance performance improvement as it is
shared with key audiences.

How are we doing? Health care organizations need to know. Their performance against established benchmarks and targets of desired performance is important information that drives performance improvement efforts. These elements of performance are increasingly being presented in balanced scorecards of performance.

Kaplan and Norton (1993, 1996a, 1996b) developed the balanced scorecard as an approach to integrating and balancing measures of performance. The balanced scorecard is like a business report card for the organization. In health care it reports on how the organization is delivering the integrated components of the value equation to its customers and stakeholders (including patients and employees). The view of performance is no longer one dimensional; it is integrated, requiring collection of integrated measures of performance. The balanced scorecard links several types of performance indicators: process, structure, value, clinical, financial performance, and cost.

Health care systems require performance measures to operate their key business processes, to manage their resources, and to lead the organization in a strategic direction. Three levels of performance are monitored: strategic, diagnostic, and operational. The balanced approach links clinical outcomes and patient satisfaction to the core business strategy and financial performance of the organization. Thus this balanced approach to performance measurement incorporates the integrated components of the value equation (Figure 1.1).

In examining the value equation, we see that value cannot be calculated or described in clinical or cost terms alone. An integrated computation is required. This integration of cost and quality metrics of value is incorporated into measurement at all levels of an organization so the results will reveal how an organization is progressing toward its goals.

The first step in creating a balanced scorecard is to define the organizational objectives. Next, metrics for each objective are defined—only a few metrics for each objective. Once metrics are defined in a way that makes sense to all audiences, an organization must find ways to collect the data to measure each objective and must determine who will collect the metrics. Finding an economical and feasible way to accomplish this takes innovation and the combining of data from a variety of sources.

A Balanced Scorecard in a Large Health Care System

The executive management of a large, integrated health care system developed a balanced approach to measuring five key organizational objectives, which focused on market share, operational and clinical excellence, customer satisfaction, workforce development, and financial resources. Twenty-two strategies were identified as necessary to provide the infrastructure needed to accomplish each objective.

Each objective and strategy was assigned a measurable metric and target. Convinced that measurement motivates, the health care system adopted the mantra "provide the right care, at the right place, in the right way, at the right time, at the right price, and be able to prove it." Proving it required a balanced measurement tool that could be easily and effectively communicated to the entire organization.

The Challenge

The system's objectives and metrics—ranging from clinical quality to financial ratios—required a tool that could communicate the system's strategic vision and the balance of the objectives in addition to the progress achieved. Because this message was to be communicated to a large and diverse audience consisting of physicians, employees, customers, and stakeholders, the tool needed to be quick to read and easy to understand. The tool had to be precise but also flexible, to handle changes of objectives, strategies, or metrics without a disruption to the scorecard report. The data quest began for an ideal tool that would

- Provide a fast but comprehensive and balanced view of the organization's plan and progress from several perspectives.
- Provide an easy-to-understand graphical display of accomplishment.
- Not compromise confidentiality of highly sensitive business and clinical data

System senior management elected to use the balanced scorecard approach because it effectively met those needs.

The Approach

The radar graph depicted in Figure 13.1 was selected to represent the scorecard. Each point on the radar graph communicates one of the five corporate objectives. The two rings report accomplishment in the form of success ratios. The outer ring represents the objec-

Figure 13.1. Example of Scorecard.

Year-to-Date Progress Toward Fiscal Year Target

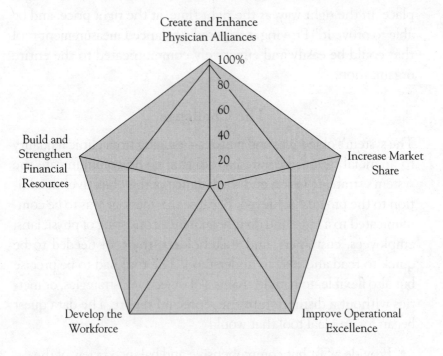

Create and Enhance
Physician Alliances

Build and
Strengthen
Financial
Resources

Increase Market
Share

Develop the
Workforce

Improve Operational
Excellence

Source: Reproduced compliments of Baylor Health Care System.

tives' targets; the inner ring shows the percentage of each target achieved. Each objective has one or more metrics. An average of the metrics' success ratios is shown for objectives that have multiple metrics. Reporting progress as a percentage of the target protects confidentiality of sensitive data and focuses on progress achieved and opportunity remaining.

The scorecard proved to be a valuable tool and needed to be efficiently communicated. Once again, the size, diversity, and geographical location of the audience were a communication challenge. The scorecard is published quarterly in the newsletters and publications of the health care system, but the most effective publication of the scorecard is on the organization's intranet.

Publishing the scorecard via the intranet has proved especially effective because it reaches a wide audience and is available to the viewer as often as needed. It also promotes continuing education, as viewers are able to access additional information such as definitions, the champions of the objectives and strategies, and the metrics for each objective and strategy. Viewers who have been granted access can drill down to secured screens that contain more specific and sensitive performance data. Access is granted on a need-to-know basis in accordance with the organization's data access policy.

The Lessons Learned

Defining the objectives and strategies and collecting the data to measure their achievement was basic to the successful generation of the balanced scorecard. Due to the diversity of the audience for the scorecard, it was important to define the objectives and strategies with as much precision as possible, using familiar terminology and avoiding buzzwords. Owners of the objectives and strategies identified metrics appropriate for measuring accomplishment and determined realistic but aggressive targets.

The level of integrated health care organization data required for balanced scorecard reporting may not be readily or easily available. It is tempting to refrain from reporting a metric until the infrastructure is in place, but a small number of good data is better than a large number of questionable data. The need for clinically robust information systems that could provide risk-adjusted, comparative clinical quality metrics for the balanced scorecard added impetus to the organization's quest for a clinical data model to support performance improvement.

Identifying appropriate indicators for each metric is the basis for the success of the entire process. It is critical that those who will actually be collecting the data define up front the process for obtaining and reporting each metric. The challenge associated with data collection of various dimensions of performance was twofold: it required integration of information from several sources in the health care system, and it required coordination of data supplied at various times. The system met this challenge by developing a reporting process in which data submitters are responsible for verifying data accuracy before providing the data to the scorecard coordinator. The scorecard coordinator then calculates quarterly success ratios and publishes the updated scorecard.

The senior management participates in a six-month formal review of all objectives, strategies, and metrics. This process assists in evaluating the relevance of the objectives and strategies to accomplish the system's vision and mission in the constantly changing health care environment.

Conclusion

Measuring progress with a balanced scorecard provides integration for organizational improvement efforts by establishing targets, measuring achievement toward targets, and communicating these definitions and findings to key audiences. The intent is to engage these audiences in the quest for improvement in organizational performance. Production of these balanced reports would be facilitated by integrated information systems; however, in today's environment most health care organizations must continue to rely on data from disparate sources.

The balanced scorecard is becoming an increasingly popular tool in health care. It can provide leaders with a comprehensive framework that translates an organization's strategic objectives into a coherent set of performance measures. The balanced scorecard remains an effective tool with which clinical knowledge workers and others can improve performance.

Chapter Fourteen

Creating a Climate of Discovery

Stephen Ryter

Clinicians need and want data about their
performance. However, the way the information is
prepared and presented influences their willingness
to discover performance improvement
opportunities. This chapter discusses key points in
creating a climate of discovery and proposes some
critical success factors for achieving clinician
acceptance of performance data.

When a health care organization wants to partner with clinicians
to deliver health care value, it must share integrated performance
data with them. Data may relate to services provided in the primary
care physician's office, referrals to specialists, laboratory and radio-
graphic services, inpatient and outpatient hospital services, and
prescription drugs. These data may exist in a variety of source systems. Performance may be tracked by plan, medical group, or individual practitioner. Data may also be generated from the claims
system, which indicates standard measures of utilization such as
hospital days and admissions per thousand members and average
length of stay for various general specialties such as medicine,
surgery, and obstetrics. The number of referrals per thousand members per year, to whom referrals are made, and the referral source
(physicians) are also examined.

Clinicians need data to determine opportunities for improvement, to benchmark or compare their performance to that of others, and to assess their performance on key aspects of patient care.

The Challenge

Among the challenges facing organizations that want to share data with clinicians is the methodology. Data need to be meticulously prepared. It is essential to have a clinician-friendly approach in order to reach these busy professionals. The timeliness of data is an issue. There may be a lag time between submission of claims and encounter data and their use. Other issues are the limitations of administrative data in adequately adjusting for severity; and the dependence on the accuracy and completeness of coding procedures to fully capture the clinical picture of the patient.

The Approach

Clinicians want to know how they compare with their peers. They need and want to see data about their practice. In spite of this, the news that they are not doing as well as their peers may not always be welcomed. The accuracy and equity of performance data is a sensitive issue for clinicians. The imperative for those preparing and presenting data is to ensure their accuracy, validity, and reliability and to present them in the most effective and efficient way. These steps are crucial in gaining clinician confidence.

There are factors that contribute to a climate of discovery. These are some of the critical success factors to consider in preparing data for clinicians with the goal of turning those data into information to improve care:

- *Accuracy.* Data must be as accurate as possible. Presenters should not go any further if they are not sure about data integrity. Unfortunately, when dealing with claims, the resultant data are only as good as the ICD and CPT codes entered by practitioners and providers and as the skill of manual claims processors.
- *Valuable information.* The information presented must answer questions of interest to the clinicians and offer enough benefit to them to warrant the time involved in collecting it. The

data should focus on a topic of study and those clinical and financial areas related to that topic. The presenter should avoid trying to cover too many clinical questions at one time. Skillful use of data is a critical skill in applying models of improvement. Organizations and providers need information to guide the three fundamental questions that drive improvement work (Langley, Nolan, Nolan, Norman, and Provost, 1996):

What are we trying to accomplish?

How will we know that a change is an improvement?

What changes can we make that will result in improvement?

- *Timeliness*. Clinical knowledge workers involved in real-time improvement efforts need data collected concurrently to improve care as it happens. Retrospective analyses of care patterns are also worthwhile for study of past patterns, but in any case the information should be as current as possible in order to support care improvement.

- *Clinician-friendly reports*. Data should be plotted over time and the report format should show any trends in variation. This method allows an observer to examine patterns and understand when a change occurs. The report format should help the clinician analyze the information quickly. Control charts and measures of significance are important. The presenter should give overview information and follow up with more detailed data by request.

- *Appropriate use of data*. Reports of performance improvement information should be designed for specific audiences, and care should be taken to ensure appropriate use and interpretation of data. Some organizations conceal the identity of clinicians when showing how members of a group of providers compare with each other. A report may be provided to several providers, but only the individual recipient knows which data represent him or her.

- *Severity adjustment.* Although administrative data offer practical advantages when measuring care, clinical content and data quality issues limit their usefulness in clinical assessment of care (Iezzoni, 1997). The adequacy of present administratively derived systems to adjust for differences in patients' severity of illness is a limiting factor in preparing credible clinical data (see Chapter Eight). In evaluating performance improvement data, clinicians will want to understand the difference in severity adjustment methods used with the data. The data can then be interpreted and used with the limitations in mind.

- *Educational approach.* The presenter's role is to facilitate discovery, inquiry, and learning. The proper presentation of data in understandable form helps this learning occur. If the presentation really turns data into information, it is likely to increase the motivation of the audience to do some study after the session and to comprehend where change may be needed. The analyst or other individual presenting data must thoroughly understand those data and know how the analysis was built. Successful data detectives have to be able not only to interpret what they present but also to discuss and even defend how the data were obtained. Otherwise, future efforts to engage the same clinicians may meet with little success. The presenter should be confident but not defensive. Clinicians may ask an analyst to recheck the data. A willingness to do this and work with clinicians until they feel confident in the numbers goes a long way toward establishing a partnership relationship.

- *Respect for clinicians' time.* The presenter should ensure that he or she has meaningful and relevant data before taking someone's time in a presentation. In addition, the presenter should consider starting a data presentation with the punch line rather than building to a great finish. The presenter's chance to make an impact will probably come at the outset.

Conclusion

The climate in which data are presented is a key factor in increasing a clinician's ability to effectively use data. A number of key factors have been suggested in this chapter that may encourage this collaborative climate of discovery. Each data pioneer is likely to discover more secrets of success. The identification and communication of these success factors throughout the clinical knowledge community will increase its ability to transfer and use information and turn it into knowledge that can improve care.

In the use of performance data most clinicians will be tourists and farmers of data. In some cases they may be anxious to devote time to exploring the data in iterations to discover ways to make care better. Creating this opportunity comes from establishing a climate of discovery each time data are presented. In delivering performance information, education and facilitation work best.

Chapter Fifteen

Common Themes

Collaboration and Creativity

Health care is delivered in complex communities of practice. Today's quest for data is an iterative process of query and discovery. This closing chapter summarizes the characteristics and themes seen in the data quests of emerging knowledge communities. It reviews the five common themes of a data quest and key issues for the future of the health care information processing organization.

Today's clinical knowledge worker is both pragmatist and visionary. Finding data in the clinical knowledge community is cumbersome. Turning these data into information and then into knowledge is even more challenging. But in spite of this most data quests succeed! Why?

The pressing demands of improving care today must simultaneously create the information delivery architecture vision for the future. The knowledge-driven inclinations of clinical workers enhance risk aversion and facilitate innovation. These aspirations coexist with a practical need to measure and monitor health care in response to immediate demands. The clinical knowledge community is self-organizing and adaptive. In spite of the limitations of the present turbulent health care information environment, or perhaps because of them, clinical knowledge workers use many innovative methods to find and use integrated data to measure and improve health care. Communities of practice are learning through collaboration what information is needed and what architecture best prepares the clinical community for the delivery of health care in the twenty-first century.

Clinical knowledge workers in search of performance improvement data search for and use data in a number of ways. Tourists prefer a dashboard of highly relevant information. This is shown in the development of the scorecard in Chapter Thirteen. Farmers are more inquisitive and perform drill-down queries until they can roll up, compare, or trend data that matter. Chapters Eleven and Twelve illustrate the tenacity of farmers in search of information to improve care. The case studies also demonstrate explorer behavior, where each query leads to another in an iterative process of discovery.

The cumulative effects of the complex environment described in this book coexist at a time of considerable limitations in health care information processing. The resulting challenges for clinical knowledge workers have fostered a dynamic impetus to develop new approaches to finding and using integrated data to improve care. The complexity of the present environment thus both encourages and supports the development of creativity and diffusion of innovation. Bowers in Chapter Ten describes this challenge as building a better boat while you are already far out to sea.

The preceding chapters focused on the complexity of the environment in which clinical knowledge workers are engaged, these workers' constant exchange of ideas, and their innovation and discovery. Complex issues and challenges confront clinical knowledge workers. Five common themes define their quest for health care data: collaboration, standardized vocabulary, reduction of non-value-added activity, creativity and diffusion of information, and clinical integration.

Collaboration

The clinical knowledge community is emerging in the midst of rapid technological and social change. In this environment, no one individual has an entire view of all aspects that affect patient care. The clinical knowledge worker, then, depends on the creative exchange of ideas with a variety of professionals. Exchange of information in real time also requires information architecture: an accessible knowledge base in a useful and accessible format that also ensures security and confidentiality of sensitive patient data.

The increased need for collaboration of clinical knowledge workers results from the following health care trends:

- Demand for health care value
- Internal and external demands for integrated data to ensure health care value
- Disparate islands of health care information
- Focus on the health care customer
- Integration and complexity of health care delivery systems
- Need for increased access to health care information accompanied by increased public concerns for privacy and protection of data
- Need for an increased climate of discovery to enhance the transformation of health care data to information and then to knowledge to improve care

Increased collaboration between clinical and financial stakeholders is occurring to bridge existing islands of information in order to measure the true value of care across episodes of care.

Standardized Vocabulary

Health care needs a common language with which to measure clinical value. A common lexicon and consistent data models allow comparative study of the best ways to deliver care. Efforts to integrate medical information across episodes of care and across sites of care delivery require unique patient identifiers and a common vocabulary.

A structured set of terms that facilitates precise communication still eludes the health care knowledge community. Work is ongoing in this area, and it seems likely that the information processing organization of the twenty-first century will be characterized by a more controlled and standardized vocabulary. The search for a common lexicon and measurement is characterized by the following trends:

- Collaborative initiatives to develop common indicator sets
- Evolution of integrated measures of value, which include service, cost, function, and quality
- Development of clinically robust measures to adjust data for severity
- National efforts at data standardization
- Efforts to improve data validity and normalization
- Partnerships of payers, providers, and public groups to develop acceptable measures of health care value that meet the criterion of "a few good measures"
- Use of Internet technology to communicate health care information

Reduction of Non-Value-Added Activity

The process of data discovery today is immediate, intense, dynamic, and problematic. Information must be mined from diverse, rapidly changing interactive systems and subsystems. Because searching for the right data can be time consuming and expensive, non-value-added data collection and stores must be minimized. Clinical knowledge workers, confronted with vast, uncoordinated, and inconsistent data stores, must distinguish the important from the unimportant, spend time looking only for measures of performance that really matter, and find innovative ways to bridge the islands of information. In spite of the fragmentation of the health care information needed for integrated study of care, clinical knowledge workers still manage to piece together vital pieces of information to measure important aspects of care.

Non-value-added activity is reduced in a successful data quest. Tools such as the data needs assessments, data blueprints, and well-planned data searches described in Chapter Two accomplish this. Understanding the limitations of administrative data for measuring care, as described in Chapter Eight, results in searches for new and more clinically robust methods to measure quality. When non-value-added data retrieval is eliminated, clinical knowledge workers can focus on analysis and knowledge transfer.

Creativity and Diffusion of Innovation

The many demands for easily understood measures of value provide a catalyst for the development of common measures of health care quality. Performance improvement in health care is a process of discovery. It is defining a question, finding data, and redefining the question. It is creative activity.

Clinical knowledge workers use an innovative process of self-discovery and adaptation during their data quests. The tools they use include emerging integrated architectures, data mining of existing islands of information, and development of common lexicons and clinically relevant definitions of quality. Clinical, cost, quality, and functional parameters are being aggregated in new tools, such as the data cubes described in Chapter Eleven, to move data toward knowledge to improve care.

Use of administratively based data is becoming less satisfactory to those who need to make comparisons among providers. At the same time, as administrative databases continue to be used, the collaborative clinical community learns more about which data and measures really represent quality and value. The search for common valid definitions continues, and the dialogue and its result will define information architecture and system requirements.

Clinical knowledge workers must communicate the fruits of their searches. Chapter Thirteen showed one way of communicating organizational progress to several audiences through a scorecard, and Chapter Fourteen addressed strategies for communicating with clinicians about data. While using and communicating about data, clinical knowledge workers must also protect the confidentiality of patients and ensure the security of informational systems, as described in Chapter Seven.

The clinical knowledge worker must be supported by an information processing organization that supports new kinds of interaction and transfer of knowledge. Chapter Three provided the conceptual model for this health care information processing organization, Chapter Four proposed a vision for an architecture that can help bring us into the twenty-first century, and Chapter Five presented some examples of the clinical systems available.

Clinical Integration

Measurement of broad populations of patients is necessary to understand care and what improves it. As explained in Chapter Nine, clinical integration requires integrated information and is a key driver of information integration. But the key premise of this chapter is that information is more than a tool. The process of integrating data becomes an improvement in the process of care delivery.

There are three key elements of clinical integration that accelerate clinical process improvement and integration of health care data:

- Integration of traditional quality improvement organizations into population-based cross-continuum measurement models
- Alignment of information system goals with the core business strategies of the integrated organization
- Development of clinically integrated data models

   Tools used in today's journeys of discovery include

- Data inventories

- Data needs assessments
- Clinical pathway analysis
- Clinical data standardization
- Redesigned approaches to quality management
- Models of information management that cross the care continuum
- Precise queries
- Multidimensional balanced scorecards of health care value
- Policies that protect patient confidentiality and control data access but also provide diffusion of information
- Climates of discovery and collaboration
- Clinically integrated information architecture
- Common quality measures

Into the Future: Key Issues

The demands of the evolving health care environment will create new questions and challenges for future study and innovation. Data detectives of the twenty-first century must find innovative ways to develop

- Economically feasible and clinically robust methods of severity of illness adjustment
- Standardization of data and a common lexicon
- Nationally accepted definitions of quality indicators that measure process and outcomes of care across the continuum
- Information infrastructures and architectures that support real-time analytical processing and that mirror new models of integrated care systems that measure care across the continuum
- Internet-enabled information transfer within the clinical knowledge community

- Data access and data confidentiality policies to guide clinical knowledge workers in sharing information while protecting patient privacy

Conclusion

The health care information processing organization is self-organizing and adapting. The learning organization of the twenty-first century is evolving. It will look vastly different from the information processing world of today. Components of the new information processing organization include data warehouses, operational data stores, data marts, and analytical tools. Territorialism, information hoarding, and nonstandardized environments are becoming dinosaurs, giving way to a new information ecosystem.

Clinical knowledge workers on data quests are often the early adopters of this new information environment and demand efficient access to high-quality information.

The health care information processing organization of the future will possess inherent creativity and innovation and will create vast social change in the clinical knowledge community. It will be an exciting journey.

References

Appavu, S. I. (1997). *Analysis of unique patient identifier options* (Final Report, Part Four). Available: www.ncvhs.hhs.gov/app4.htm.

Bergman, R. (1994). Getting the goods on guidelines. *Hospitals and Health Networks, 68*(20), 70–74.

Broverman, C. A. (1999). Standards for clinical decision support systems. *Journal of Healthcare Information Management, 13*(2), 23–31.

Brunner, R., & Brewer, C. (1977). *Organized complexity: Empirical theories on political development.* New York: Free Press.

Conrad, D. A. (1993). Coordinating patient care services in regional health care systems: The challenge of clinical integration. *Hospitals and Health Services Administration, 38*(4), 491–508.

Coyne, J. (1993). Assessing the financial performance of health maintenance organizations: Tools and techniques. *Managed Care Quarterly, 1,* 63.

Demarest, M. (1994, July). Data marts. *DBMS.*

Drucker, P. (1985). *Innovation and entrepreneurship.* New York: HarperCollins.

Electronic Frontier Foundation. (1993). *Protecting privacy in computerized medical information* (U.S. Office of Technology Assessment report). Available: www.eff.org/pub/Privacy/Medical/1993_ota_medical_privacy.report.

Gilbreath, R., Nelson, M., Schilp, J., & Burch, J. (1996). Determining the financial return on the study investment. In Spath, P. (ed.), *Medical effectiveness and outcomes management.* Chicago: American Hospital Publishing.

Horn, S., & Hopkins, D. (1994). *Clinical practice improvement.* New York: Faulkner and Gray.

Iezzoni, L. I. (1997). Assessing quality using administrative data. *Annals of Internal Medicine, 127,* 666–674.

Inmon, W. (1993). *Building the data warehouse.* New York: Wiley.

Inmon, W., Imhoff, C., & Battas, G. (1995). *Building the operational data store.* New York: Wiley.

Inmon, W., Imhoff, C., & Sousa, R. (1998). *Corporate information factory.* New York: Wiley Computer.

Joint Commission on Accreditation of Healthcare Organizations. (1999). *Data quality principles*. Available: http://wwwa.jcaho.org/perfmeas/ dqprinc.html.

Joint Commission on Accreditation of Healthcare Organizations. (1999). *Performance measures: Glossary of terms*. Available: http://wwwa.jcaho.org/ perfmeas.glossry.html.

Kaplan, R. S., & Norton, D. P. (1993). Putting the balanced scorecard to work. *Harvard Business Review, 71*(5), 134–147.

Kaplan, R., & Norton, D. (1996a). *The balanced scorecard*. Boston: Harvard Business School Press.

Kaplan, R. S., & Norton, D. P. (1996b). Using the balanced scorecard as a strategic management system. *Harvard Business Review, 74*(1), 75–85.

Kimball, R. (1996). *The data warehouse toolkit*. New York: Wiley.

Langley, G., Nolan, K., Nolan, T., Norman, C., and Provost, L. (1996). *The improvement guide*. San Francisco: Jossey-Bass, p. 3.

Longo, D. (1988). Preface. In B. James, *Quality management for health care delivery*. Chicago: Hospital Research and Education Trust of the American Hospital Association.

Luttman, R., Siren, P., & Laffel, G. (1994). Assessing organizational performance. *Quality Management in Health Care, 2*, 44.

Manion, J., Lorimer, W., & Leander, W. (1996). *Team based health care organizations: Blueprint for success*. Gaithersburg, MD: Aspen.

Manville, B., & Foote, N. (1996a). Harvest your workers' knowledge. *Datamation*.

Manville, B., & Foote, N. (1996b). Strategy as if knowledge mattered. *Fast Company*.

Maxwell, C., Zeigenfuss, J., & Chisholm, R. (1993). Beyond quality improvement teams: Sociotechnical systems theory and self-directed work teams. *Quality Management in Health Care, 1*(2), 59-67.

McGlynn, E., Damberg, C., Kerr, E., & Shenker, E. (1998). Building an integrated information system. Available: www.chmis.org/qmas/chds1.html.

National Research Council. (1997). *For the record: Protecting electronic health information*. Washington, DC: National Academy Press.

Office of Technology Assessment. U.S. Congress. (1994). *Identifying health technologies that work: Searching for evidence* (OTA-H–608). Washington, DC: U.S. Government Printing Office.

Pava, C. (1986). Redesigning sociotechnical systems design: Concepts and methods for the '90s. *Journal of Applied Behavioral Science, 22*, 201.

Raden, N. (1995, October). Data data everywhere. *Information Week*.

Rogers, E. (1995). *Diffusion of innovations* (4th ed.). New York: Free Press.

Ruffin, M. (1995, July). Capitation and informatics. *Physician Executive, 21*, 21.

Salem-Schatz, S., Moore, G., Rucker, M., & Pearson, S. (1994, September). The case-mix adjustment in practice profiling: When good apples look bad. *Journal of the American Medical Association, 272*, 871–921.

Sharp, L., & Priesmeyer, H. (1995). Tutorial: Chaos theory—A primer for healthcare. *Quality Management in Healthcare, 3*, 71–86.

Shortell, S. M., Gillies, R. R., Anderson, D. A., Erickson, K. M., & Mitchell, J. B. (1996). *Remaking health care in America.* San Francisco: Jossey-Bass.

Shortell, S. M., Gillies, R. R., Anderson, D. A., Mitchell, J. B., & Morgan, K. L. (1993). Creating organized delivery systems: The barriers and facilitators. *Hospitals and Health Services Administration, 38*(4), 447–466.

Tonges, M. (1998). *Clinical integration: Strategies and practices for organized delivery systems.* San Francisco: Jossey-Bass.

U.S. Department of Health and Human Services. (1997). *Confidentiality of individually-identifiable health information: Recommendations of the secretary of Health and Human Services.* Available: http://aspe.os.dhhs.gov/admnsimp/pvcrec.htm.

U.S. Department of Health and Human Services (n.d). Available: http://aspe.os.dhhs.gov/admnsimp/pvcrec2.htm.

Glossary

ADT—admissions, discharge, transfer.

AHCPR—Agency for Health Care Policy and Research.

Appropriateness—"the degree to which the care provided is relevant to the patient's clinical needs, given the current state of knowledge" (Joint Commission on Accreditation of Healthcare Organizations [JCAHO], 1999).

ARTEMIS—Advanced Research Testbed for Medical Informatics.

BHCS—Baylor Health Care System.

BUMC—Baylor University Medical Center.

CABG—Coronary artery bypass graft.

Care coordination—an examination of all the relevant aspects that affect patient choice (psychological, social, economic, medical, and so forth) and a consideration of medical necessity in order to optimize the placement of the patient with the right provider, in the right setting, and ultimately at the right intensity of level of care.

Care management—the application of preventive and health maintenance interventions that improve the target population's health.

Clinical effectiveness—a measure of the effects and efficiency of a delivery process or intervention in a target population.

Clinical integration—the extent to which patient care activities are coordinated across the continuum of care to increase the probability of maximum value to the patient.

Clinical pathway—a tool to organize and time interdisciplinary team interventions for a patient with a particular case type, subset, or condition (Bergman, 1994).

Communities of practice—"self-organizing, regulating, informal networks of workers doing similar work, bound to one another through exposure to a common set of problems, embodying a store of knowledge in the common pursuit of solutions . . . driven by a mutual obligation to assist one another and having a sense of group accountability" (Manville & Foote, 1996b).

Continuous quality improvement—a philosophy of management that strives to improve performance through exclusion of poor quality during production or delivery of the service, in contrast to relying on correcting problems at a later date.

CPR—computerized patient records.

CPT—current procedural terminology.

CQI—continuous quality improvement.

CQIP—continuous quality improvement project.

Data element—"a discrete piece of data, such as patient birth date or principle diagnosis code" (JCAHO, 1999).

Data mart—the "corner information store of the online enterprise within the integrated structure of the data warehouse (enterprise data store)" (Demarest, 1994).

Data mining—the process of discovering meaningful associations, patterns, and trends by scrutinizing large amounts of historical data stored in data warehouses, using various pattern recognition, statistical, and visualization techniques.

Data quest—The iterative process of query and discovery used by clinical knowledge workers to obtain data about the processes and outcomes of health care.

Data source—"a primary source used for data collection" (JCAHO, 1999).

Data warehouse—a "subject oriented, integrated, non-volatile, time variant collection of data in support of management decisions" (Inmon, 1993).

DDW—dimensional data warehouse.

Demand management—a facet of care management that implements interventions in the general population and in patients in certain disease states in order to improve patient access to care intentionally and at an earlier time in the disease process, with the goal of reducing the demand that occurs in patients without the intervention.

Diffusion in organizations—"the process by which an innovation is communicated through certain channels over time among the members of a social system or organization" (Rogers, 1995).

Disease management—a facet of care management that focuses on certain high-risk disease states with programmatic interventions designed to improve access and quality and reduce unnecessary costs.

DRG—diagnosis related group.

DSS—decision support system.

DWMS—data warehouse management system.

EDI—electronic data interchange.

Efficiency—"the relationship between the results of care (outcomes) and the resources used to deliver the care" (JCAHO, 1999).

Emergent control—a system in which solutions come forth from the fringes of the organization.

EU—European Union.

Explorers—data seekers who insist on ad hoc query capability and rely heavily on iteration. Explorers will devote many hours to the investigation of a hunch and will not be deterred by failure to show significance. They love the hunt of investigation and will be satisfied if they only occasionally have success (Inmon, Imhoff, & Sousa, 1998).

Farmers—data seekers who are inquisitive and are willing to work hard and long to get results but who still prefer a high return on the time invested in the analysis. Farmers are satisfied most of the time by preformatted queries with standard drill down, roll up, comparison, and trending detail (Inmon, Imhoff, & Sousa, 1998).

FTE—full-time equivalent.

Functional status—levels of health status factors including physical functioning, role functioning due to physical health problems, bodily pain, general health perceptions, vitality, social functioning, role disability due to emotional problems, and general mental health.

HCFA—Health Care Financing Administration.

HEDIS—Health Plan Employer Data and Information Set.

HIM—health information management.

HIMSS—Healthcare Information and Management Systems Society.

HIPAA—Health Insurance Portability and Accountability Act.

HL7—Health Level Seven, a formatting and protocol standard.

HSS—U.S. Department of Health and Human Services.

ICD-9—International Classification of Diseases—ninth revision.

IPA—independent practice association.

JCAHO—Joint Commission on Accreditation of Healthcare Organizations.

Knowledge worker—a relational worker who has access to and uses the corporate knowledge base to make better operational decisions, usually in real time (Drucker, 1985).

LAN—local area network.

Medical management—the set of interventions applied in order to improve the health of the target population and mitigate the financial risk inherent in that population for health care costs.

MOLAP—multidimensional on-line analytical processing.

NCQA—National Committee for Quality Assurance.

ODS—operational data store.

OLAP—on-line analytical processing.

OLTP—on-line transaction processing.

Operational data store—a collection of data that is subject oriented, integrated, and volatile and reflects a current or near current collection of data in support of operational workers for immediate or near-term decision making.

Outcome measure—"a measure that indicates the result of the performance (or nonperformance) of a function or process" (JCAHO, 1999).

PC—personal computer.

PCCO—provider-sponsored coordinated care organization.

PDCA—plan, do, check, act, the continuous improvement cycle.

Performance improvement—a process of diligently examining current practices, applying process interventions, and measuring progress toward an objective level of achievement.

Performance measure—"a quantitative tool (for example rate, ratio, index, or percentage) that measures an organization's performance in relation to a specified outcome or process" (JCAHO, 1999).

Physician and provider profiles—measures of individual performance and variation from the benchmark of a key clinical parameter.

Process measure—a measure that focuses on an interrelated series of events, activities, actions, mechanisms, or steps that transform inputs into outputs. "A process measure focuses on a process that leads to a certain outcome, meaning that a scientific basis exists for believing that the process, when executed well, will increase the likelihood of achieving a desired outcome" (JCAHO, 1999).

PTCA—percutaneous transluminal coronary angioplasty.

QA—quality assurance.

RAID—redundant array of inexpensive disks.

RDBMS—relational database management system.

Reliability—"the ability of a measure to accurately and consistently identify the elements it was designed to identify across multiple health care settings" (JCAHO, 1999).

RFI—request for information.

RFP—request for proposal.

ROLAP—relational on-line analytical processing.

Satisfaction measures—"measures that address the extent to which patients or enrollees and practitioners or purchasers perceive their needs to be met" (JCAHO, 1999).

SDLC—systems development life cycle.

Severity of illness classification—"seriousness or stage of illness at the time of the observation or treatment" (JCAHO, 1999).

SF 36—Short Form 36, a thirty-six-item health status questionnaire.

SMR—structured medical record.

SQL—structured query language.

Tourists—data seekers who prefer a dashboard of highly relevant, readily accessible, summary information (Inmon, Imhoff, & Sousa, 1998).

UM—utilization management.

UMLS—Unified Medical Language System.

Validity—"ability to identify improvement opportunities in the quality of care; demonstration that the use of the measure results in improvement in outcomes or quality of care" (JCAHO, 1999). A valid measure measures what it is supposed to measure.

WAN—wide area network.

Index

Tonges, M., 7
Tourists, 50, 54, 110, 202
Trade-offs, between quality and cost, 88
Transaction-level detail, importance of, 115
Transcribed reports, 163–164, 165
Transcription system, 163–165, 170
Trending, 46, 49, 50, 53, 65, 66; farmers and, 51, 202
Trends, data, 5, 36–37, 69, 90, 197
Trust-building, 116

U

UB92 hospital discharge forms, 110
U.S. Code, vol. 42, sec. 290dd–2, 130
U.S. Code, vol. 42, secs. 1301 et seq., part C, secs. 1171–1175 (Subtitle F, Administrative Simplification), 132
U.S. Department of Health and Human Services (HHS), secretary of, recommendations by, 131–135, 136, 138, 139
Updates, and e-mail, 109
Utilization, 81, 115, 177, 178
Utilization data, 5, 9, 81
Utilization management, 58, 91, 93, 156, 157, 167–170
Utilization measures, 195
Utilization review, 58, 78

V

Validity, 6, 17, 18, 64, 181; efforts to improve, 204; standards for, 157–158
Value, 3, 4, 8, 76; creating, 36; delineation of, 27; documenting, 4
Value equation, 9, 16–17, 60, 92; and balanced scorecards, 189, 190; defined, 4, 5, 88
Value improvement, 88

Value measures, 11, 16, 190
Variance capture system, 184
Variance data, 185
Variation: overestimation of, 74; trends in, 197
Vendor evaluation & selection, 60, 84–85, 150
Videoconferencing, 77
Vision alignment, 116
Vocabulary, standard, using, 64
Vocabulary standardization, 28, 33, 205, 207; and abstracts, 92; catalyst for, 148; for data integration, 51, 203–204; in data transformation, 46; requiring, 58; and severity systems, 150–151; standards for, 40
Voice recognition, 73

W

Walker, J., 189
WAN, use of, 163, 170, 176
Web-based architectures, 70
Weblink technology, 166, 170
Websites, 10, 139
Weed, L., 73
"When Good Apples Look Bad" (Salem-Schatz, Moore, Rucker, & Pearson), 74
Windows applications, 163, 165
Worker empowerment, 90
Worker's Compensation, 81
Workflow, and self-directed work teams, 107
Workflow automation and decision support, 47, 58, 69, 72
Workflow metaphor, 72

Z

Zeigenfuss, J., 98